Hemodynamic Monitoring in the Diagnosis and Management of Heart Failure

Guest Editors

WILLIAM T. ABRAHAM, MD, FACP, FACC, FAHA
RAGAVENDRA R. BALIGA, MD, MBA

HEART FAILURE CLINICS

www.heartfailure.theclinics.com

Consulting Editors
RAGAVENDRA R. BALIGA, MD, MBA
JAMES B. YOUNG, MD

Founding Editor
JAGAT NARULA, MD, PhD

April 2009 • Volume 5 • Number 2

SAUNDERS an imprint of ELSEVIER, Inc.

ERIN K. DONAHO, RN, BSN
Heart Failure Center, St. Luke's Episcopal Institute–Texas Heart Institute, Houston, Texas

MARK H. DRAZNER, MD, MSc
Medical Director, Heart Failure and Cardiac Transplantation, University of Texas Southwestern Medical Center, Department of Internal Medicine, Division of Cardiology, Dallas, Texas

GARRIE J. HAAS, MD
Professor of Internal Medicine and Director of Cardiovascular Clinical and Translational Research Organization, Division of Cardiovascular Medicine, Department of Internal Medicine, The Ohio State University Medical Center, Davis Heart/Lung Research Institute, Columbus, Ohio

RAMI KAHWASH, MD
Fellow in Advanced Heart Failure and Cardiac Resynchronization Therapy, Division of Cardiovascular Medicine, The Ohio State University, Davis Heart/Lung Research Institute, Columbus, Ohio

DAVID A. KASS, MD
Abraham and Virginia Weiss Professor of Cardiology, Division of Cardiology, Department of Medicine, Johns Hopkins Medical Institutions, Baltimore, Maryland

CARL V. LEIER, MD
The James W. Overstreet Professor of Internal Medicine, Division of Cardiovascular Medicine, Department of Internal Medicine, The Ohio State University, Davis Heart/Lung Research Institute; and Professor, Department of Pharmacology, The Ohio State University Medical Center, Columbus, Ohio

ALAN S. MAISEL, MD
Professor of Medicine, Division of Cardiology, University of California San Diego Medical Center; and Veterans Affairs Medical Center, San Diego, California

LESLIE MILLER, MD
Walters Chair of Cardiovascular Medicine and Director of Cardiology Programs, Washington Hospital Center and Georgetown University Hospital, Washington, DC

TED PLAPPERT, CVT
Division of Cardiology, Department of Medicine, University of Pennsylvania Medical Center, Philadelphia, Pennsylvania

HIND RAHMOUNI, MD
Division of Cardiology, Department of Medicine, University of Pennsylvania Medical Center, Philadelphia, Pennsylvania

JEAN-PAUL SCHMID, MD
Centro Cardiologico Monzino, IRCCS, Instituto di Cardiologia, University of Milan, Milan, Italy; Cardiovascular Prevention and Rehabilitation, Department of Cardiology, Bern University Hospital, University of Bern, Bern, Switzerland

ISH SINGLA, MD
Instructor, Division of Cardiovascular Diseases, Department of Medicine, University of Alabama at Birmingham, Birmingham, Alabama

MARTIN G. ST. JOHN SUTTON, MBBS, FRCP
John Bryfogle Professor of Cardiovascular Diseases, Division of Cardiology, Department of Medicine, University of Pennsylvania Medical Center, Philadelphia, Pennsylvania

JOSÉ A. TALLAJ, MD
Associate Professor, Division of Cardiovascular Diseases, Department of Medicine, University of Alabama at Birmingham; and Birmingham Veterans Affairs Medical Center, Birmingham, Alabama

PAM R. TAUB, MD
Division of Cardiology, University of California San Diego Medical Center, San Diego, California

ROBIN J. TRUPP, PhD, RN, NP
The Ohio State University, College of Nursing, Columbus, Ohio

JUSTIN M. VADER, MD
University of Texas Southwestern Medical Center, Dallas, Texas

CLYDE W. YANCY, MD
Medical Director, Baylor Heart and Vascular Institute; and Chief of Cardiothoracic Transplantation, Division of Cardiothoracic Transplantation, Baylor University Medical Center, Dallas, Texas

Contributors

PAM R. TAUB, MD
Division of Cardiology, University of California
San Diego Medical Center, San Diego,
California

ROBIN J. TRUPP, PhD, RN, NP
The Ohio State University, College of Nursing,
Columbus, Ohio

JUSTIN M. YADER, MD
University of Texas Southwestern Medical
Center, Dallas, Texas

CLYDE W. YANCY, MD
Medical Director, Baylor Heart and Vascular
Institute; and Chief of Cardiothoracic
Transplantation, Division of Cardiothoracic
Transplantation, Baylor University Medical
Center, Dallas, Texas

Contents

Heart failure is a clinical syndrome defined by the presence of characteristic signs and symptoms. History taking and physical examination have particular utility in assessing patients who have heart failure. In recent years the validity of conventional signs and symptoms of heart failure has been tested in large population studies and in clinical trials, providing an evidence basis for their utility in the clinical assessment of the patient who has known or suspected heart failure. There also has been progress in characterizing the process of acute decompensation from a previously chronic stable state. This article addresses the usefulness of signs and symptoms and daily weights in the assessment and management of patients who have heart failure.

Impedance cardiography technology, along with recent advances in the impedance cardiography (ICG) device, has become a provocative but not yet proven noninvasive alternative to invasive hemodynamic measurements. The results from stroke volume and cardiac output measurements by ICG show reasonably accurate correlation to the values calculated from direct measurements from pulmonary artery catheters. ICG may be a useful adjunct to clinical judgment for heart failure patients. The available data would not yet support supplanting invasive hemodynamic assessment in the critical care setting with ICG. Future studies and advances in technology are expected to improve impedance cardiography, thus broadening its clinical applications. Ongoing research must confirm the precise benefits of this information for ICG monitoring to become a standard assessment in heart failure.

Pulmonary congestion can be challenging to diagnose because of nonspecific symptoms and the blunt nature of physical examination and radiographic findings. Assessing for euvolemia following treatment of congestion also can be difficult but can improve both the inpatient and outpatient care of patients who have heart failure. Tools such as the natriuretic peptides are important adjuncts to the physical

examination and chest radiographs and often obviate the need for invasive hemodynamic assessment.

Assessment of Left Ventricular Systolic Function by Echocardiography   177

Martin G. St. John Sutton, Ted Plappert, and Hind Rahmouni

Echocardiography serves an extremely important role in the diagnosis and management of patients with heart failure. The various stages of structural and functional
changes that constitute progressive left ventricle remodeling have all been characterized by two-dimensional echocardiography. In addition, echocardiography has
defined the transition from compensated hypertrophy to left ventricle dilatation
and progression to end-stage heart failure. Echocardiography has also played an
important role in clinical heart failure trials of β-adrenergic blocking agents and
angiotensin-converting enzyme inhibitors and angiotensin receptor blockers and
demonstrated their efficacy in heart failure.

The Role of Echocardiography in Hemodynamic Assessment in Heart Failure   191

Jacob Abraham and Theodore P. Abraham

Echocardiography now is recommended as the most useful diagnostic test for
routine evaluation and management of heart failure. This article reviews the role of
echocardiography (M-mode, two-dimensional, spectral, and tissue Doppler) for
qualitative and quantitative hemodynamic assessment of the patient who has heart
failure. It highlights the echocardiographic parameters that have the most diagnostic
and/or prognostic relevance for patients who have advanced heart failure. The
importance of right heart failure and heart failure with preserved ejection fraction
is increasingly recognized, and therefore the echocardiographic evaluation of these
conditions is emphasized also.

Noninvasive Measurement of Cardiac Output During Exercise by Inert Gas
Rebreathing Technique   209

Gaia Cattadori, Jean-Paul Schmid, and Piergiuseppe Agostoni

Reduced exercise tolerance and dyspnea during exercise are hallmarks of heart failure syndrome. Exercise capacity and various parameters of cardiopulmonary
response to exercise are of important prognostic value. All the available parameters
only indirectly reflect left ventricular dysfunction and hemodynamic adaptation to an
increased demand. Noninvasive assessment of cardiac output, especially during an
incremental exercise stress test, would allow the direct measure of cardiac reserve
and may become the gold standard for prognostic evaluation in the future.

Invasive Hemodynamic Assessment in Heart Failure   217

Barry A. Borlaug and David A. Kass

Routine cardiac catheterization provides data on left heart, right heart, systemic and
pulmonary arterial pressures, vascular resistances, cardiac output, and ejection
fraction. These data are often then applied as markers of cardiac preload, afterload,
and global function, although each of these parameters reflects more complex interactions between the heart and its internal and external loads. This article reviews
more specific gold standard assessments of ventricular and arterial properties,
and how these relate to the parameters reported and utilized in practice, and then

discusses the re-emerging importance of invasive hemodynamics in the assessment and management of heart failure.

This article addresses a question that the authors consider to be somewhat rhetorical: are hemodynamic parameters predictors of mortality? It reviews the specific hemodynamic abnormalities and pathophysiologic consequences distinctive to the patient who has decompensation and addresses the data that implicate abnormal hemodynamics as a treatment target associated with increased mortality. The focus is on patients who have decompensated heart failure, defined as left ventricular systolic dysfunction and an acute, subacute, or gradual worsening of symptoms while receiving optimal medical therapy.

The pulmonary artery catheter will likely earn a place in the history of medicine as one of the most useful tools that shaped our understanding and management of various diseases. An intense assessment of its application in nonacute and nonshock decompensated heart failure has been provided by the ESCAPE trial, a landmark investigation that showed an overall neutral impact of pulmonary artery catheter–guided therapy over therapy guided by clinical evaluation and judgment alone. The current guidelines reserve the use of a pulmonary artery catheter for the management of refractory heart failure and select conditions. The pulmonary artery catheter remains a useful instrument in clinical situations when clinical and laboratory assessment alone is insufficient in establishing the diagnosis and pathophysiologic condition, and in guiding effective, safe therapy.

To precisely deliver appropriate therapy, cardiac resynchronization therapy devices track vast amounts of physiologic information. This information may be useful in monitoring heart failure patients and may provide meaningful insight into physiologic stability of volume status, activity, and cardiac electrophysiology. It is presumed that frequent monitoring of heart failure patients reduces the morbidity of heart failure by providing information early on so that measures can be taken to prevent congestion leading to acute decompensation. Until recently, however, frequent monitoring required face-to-face encounters in an office setting. Acquisition of device-based diagnostic information is now possible with Internet-based information systems. This article reviews the nature of device-based diagnostic information, examines how its clinical use can be justified, and makes suggestions for work flow that can make information from implanted devices useful in a clinical setting.

The evaluation and management of volume status in patients with heart failure is a challenge for most clinicians. In addition, such an evaluation is possible only during a personal clinician–patient interface. The ability to acquire hemodynamic data continuously with the help of implanted devices with remote monitoring capability can provide early warning of heart failure decompensation and thus may aid in preventing hospitalizations for heart failure. The data obtained also may improve the understanding of the disease process. It is important for the clinician treating patients who have heart failure to become acquainted with this type of technology and learn to interpret and use these data appropriately. This article reviews the implantable hemodynamics monitors currently available.

Managing patients who have heart failure is challenging and requires the integration of inpatient and outpatient care. Until evidence from clinical trials of implantable hemodynamic monitors (IHMs) is available and approval from the Food and Drug Administration is received, the best available model seems to be telemonitoring in conjunction with a comprehensive heart failure disease management program. A number of issues, including established processes for data review and interpretation, must be addressed before IHMs are widely adopted and accepted. Nurses, as the most frequent and common contact for patients, have the ability and opportunity to lead this change.

Heart Failure Clinics

THE CLINICS ARE NOW AVAILABLE ONLINE!

Access your subscription at:
www.theclinics.com

Preface

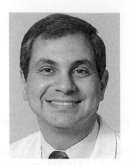 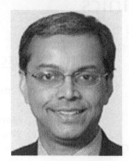

William T. Abraham, MD, FACP, FACC, FAHA   Ragavendra R. Baliga, MD, MBA

Guest Editors

Elevated ventricular filling pressures, which typically begin rising weeks before hospitalization, play a major role in the underlying pathophysiology of acute decompensated heart failure. Thus, ambulatory hemodynamic monitoring may prove to be helpful in preventing and treating episodes of heart failure decompensation. An increased understanding of the tools available for monitoring the clinical status of heart failure should allow us to develop more effective therapy and prevention strategies for all patients who have chronic and acutely decompensated heart failure.

This special issue of *Heart Failure Clinics* is dedicated to the discussion of the role of hemodynamic monitoring of heart failure. The articles in the issue range from the clinical evaluation of hemodynamics, to a nursing perspective on hemodynamic monitoring, to future technologies that should play an important role in the management of chronic and acutely decompensated heart failure.

We hope that these articles, which were authored by leading experts in the field, are not only informative but also will provide stimulus for further research that will improve the future management of heart failure.

William T. Abraham, MD, FACP, FACC, FAHA
The Ohio State University
Columbus, OH, USA

Ragavendra R. Baliga, MD, MBA
The Ohio State University
Columbus, OH, USA

E-mail addresses:
William.Abraham@osumc.edu (W.T. Abraham)
Ragavendra.Baliga@osumc.edu (R.R. Baliga)

Heart Failure Clin 5 (2009) xv
doi:10.1016/j.htc.2008.12.004
1551-7136/08/$ – see front matter © 2009 Elsevier Inc. All rights reserved.

Editorial

Bench to Bedside to Home: Homing-in on Therapy that Begins at Home

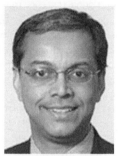 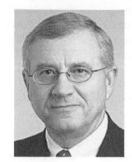

Ragavendra R. Baliga, MD, MBA   James B. Young, MD
Consulting Editors

The management of acute decompensated heart failure has traditionally focused on the treatment of patients within the four walls of hospitals. Patients who have manifest heart failure typically have pulmonary congestion, and, in some patients, decreased cardiac output with hypoperfusion may dominate the presentation. Traditionally, right heart catheterization was used to determine and monitor filling pressures to better manage heart failure, but studies from the Evaluation Study of Congestive Heart Failure and Pulmonary Artery Catheterization Effectiveness (ESCAPE) trial suggested that the risk to benefit ratio of this procedure was such that the incremental value of routine right heart catheterization with hemodynamic evaluation came into question.[1] The quest for early detection of pulmonary congestion resulted in the development of several noninvasive modalities for hemodynamic evaluation. The value of these modalities should increase if rehospitalization rates decrease. This means that the focus of management of heart failure begins at home.

Better understanding of the pathogenesis of heart failure suggests that hemodynamic impairment in this syndrome is not limited to the perturbation of cardiac filling pressures but also encompasses alternations in the entire vascular system.[2,3] The quest for early detection of acute decompensated heart failure would, therefore, require technology that would detect these changes both in the heart and the vascular system. The detection of pulmonary congestion[4] requires determination of left-sided filling pressures, such as atrial pressure, pulmonary capillary wedge pressure, and left ventricular end-diastolic pressure. The detection of right-sided heart failure requires measurement of right-sided filling pressures, such as central venous pressure, particularly in the setting of hypotension. Current noninvasive modalities, including implantable hemodynamic monitors, typically detect pressures in the right heart, which are then used to estimate left-sided filling pressures.[5,6] The new paradigm that "acute vascular failure" or "stiff central arteries" contributes to decompensated heart failure should stimulate the development of new technologies to detect hemodynamic changes in the central arteries, including the aorta.[2,3]

In this issue, William T. Abraham, MD, and one of us invited a world-class team of leading experts in the field of cardiovascular hemodynamics to elaborate on the current relevance of hemodynamics in the management of acute decompensated heart failure (ADHF). The first step is early detection of heart failure and these new disruptive technologies provide us with details of predictors of ADHF, such as measures of filling pressures,[4] weight gain due to edema, and shortness of breath. The next step would be the ability to deliver

Heart Failure Clin 5 (2009) xiii–xiv
doi:10.1016/j.hfc.2008.12.003
1551-7136/08/$ – see front matter

therapy in real-time to be effective. The latter would require the development of a comprehensive disease management program that is patient-centric. This is particularly important as more and more elderly patients develop heart failure.[7] Development of all technologies starts at the bench before it arrives at the bedside. Although the management of ADHF is at the hospital bedside, prevention of symptomatic progression is at home.[8] Preventive strategies, such as diminution of fluid overload, interdiction of medication, nontreatment of cardiac arrhythmias, and myocardial ischemia, have shown to be beneficial in heart failure.[9,10] All of these approaches could be modified, augmented, or triggered based on "early warning" information that might be at hand. We hope that this issue will provoke thought and more research that will focus on developing technologies, algorithms, disease-management programs, and therapies that start at home—it is time to "home-in" on the domiciliary management of heart failure.

Ragavendra R. Baliga, MD, MBA
The Ohio State University
Columbus, OH, USA

James B. Young, MD
Division of Medicine
Lerner College of Medicine
Cleveland Clinic
Cleveland, OH, USA

E-mail addresses:
Ragavendra.Baliga@osumc.edu (R.R. Baliga)
YOUNGJ@ccf.org (J.B. Young)

REFERENCES

1. Binanay C, Califf RM, Hasselblad V, et al. Evaluation study of congestive heart failure and pulmonary artery catheterization effectiveness: the ESCAPE trial. JAMA 2005;294(13):1625–33.
2. Baliga RR, Young JB. "Stiff central arteries" syndrome: does a weak heart really stiff the kidney? Heart Fail Clin 2008;4(4):ix–xii.
3. Cotter G, Felker GM, Adams KF, et al. The pathophysiology of acute heart failure—is it all about fluid accumulation? Am Heart J 2008;155(1):9–18.
4. Zile MR, Bennett TD, St. John Sutton M, et al. Transition from chronic compensated to acute decompensated heart failure: pathophysiological insights obtained from continuous monitoring of intracardiac pressures. Circulation 2008;118(14):1433–41.
5. Bourge RC, Abraham WT, Adamson PB, et al. Randomized controlled trial of an implantable continuous hemodynamic monitor in patients with advanced heart failure: the COMPASS-HF study. J Am Coll Cardiol 2008;51(11):1073–9.
6. Zile MR, Bourge RC, Bennett TD, et al. Application of implantable hemodynamic monitoring in the management of patients with diastolic heart failure: a subgroup analysis of the COMPASS-HF trial. J Card Fail 2008;14(10):816–23.
7. Rosamond W, Flegal K, Furie K, et al. Heart disease and stroke statistics–2008 update: a report from the American Heart Association Statistics Committee and Stroke Statistics Subcommittee. Circulation 2008;117(4):e25–146.
8. Stewart S, Pearson S, Horowitz JD. Effects of a home-based intervention among patients with congestive heart failure discharged from acute hospital care. Arch Intern Med 1998;158(10):1067–72.
9. Stewart S, Vandenbroek AJ, Pearson S, et al. Prolonged beneficial effects of a home-based intervention on unplanned readmissions and mortality among patients with congestive heart failure. Arch Intern Med 1999;159(3):257–61.
10. Rondinini L, Coceani M, Borelli G, et al. Survival and hospitalization in a nurse-led domiciliary intervention for elderly heart failure patients. J Cardiovasc Med (Hagerstown) 2008;9(5):470–5.

Clinical Assessment of Heart Failure: Utility of Symptoms, Signs, and Daily Weights

Justin M. Vader, MD, Mark H. Drazner, MD, MSc*

KEYWORDS

- Heart failure • Diagnosis • Prognosis
- Disease management • History • Physical examination

Heart failure affects an estimated 5.8 million people, represents the primary discharge diagnosis of more than 1 million annual hospitalizations, and accounts for an estimated annual health care cost of $34.8 billion.[1] The incidence of heart failure has not decreased during the past 2 decades, although survival has improved.[2] Because the incidence of heart failure increases with age, and the oldest segments of the population in Western countries are the fastest growing of all,[3] the prevalence of heart failure will increase. Understanding the signs and symptoms of heart failure is therefore of increasing necessity.

Heart failure is a clinical syndrome defined by the presence of characteristic signs and symptoms. All major cardiology societies require the presence of symptoms for the diagnosis of heart failure, and the system used most commonly to characterize the severity of heart failure, the New York Heart Association (NYHA) classification, relies on the fundamental relationship between exertion and symptoms. History taking and physical examination form the foundation of any clinical encounter, represent an inexpensive and time-tested means to achieving an appropriate diagnosis, and have particular utility in assessing patients who have heart failure. There are, however, legitimate concerns that recently trained physicians are becoming less proficient in the performance of physical examination. Structured teaching in American postgraduate medical training is lacking, and cardiac auscultation skills among trainees are no better than among third-year medical students.[4,5] In a survey of Finnish primary practitioners, jugular vein pulsation, the basic assessment of intravascular volume status, was documented in only 3% of visits for symptomatic heart failure.[6] Meanwhile, technologies available for the assessment of cardiac performance and volume status are increasing in number, variety, and availability. The availability of these technologies and the lack of training in auscultation has created an environment in which physicians increasingly are dependent on technology to assess and manage patients. Some have expressed concerns that this change is deleterious to medical practice,[7] and others have called for a restoration of bedside medicine through structured education and skills examination.[8] In an era of evidence-based medicine, however, recent evidence overwhelmingly revolves around new and developing technologies, a situation that has the potential to usurp the role of the history and physical examination.

Fortunately, in recent years the validity of conventional signs and symptoms of heart failure has been tested in large population studies and in databases from clinical trials, providing an evidence basis for their utility in the clinical assessment of the patient who has known or suspected heart failure. There also has been progress in characterizing the process of acute decompensation of

University of Texas Southwestern Medical Center, Dallas, TX, USA
* Corresponding author. University of Texas Southwestern Medical Center, Department of Internal Medicine, Division of Cardiology, 5323 Harry Hines Blvd., Dallas, TX 75390-9047.
E-mail address: Mark.Drazner@UTSouthwestern.edu (M.H. Drazner).

Heart Failure Clin 5 (2009) 149–160
doi:10.1016/j.hfc.2008.11.001
1551-7136/08/$ – see front matter © 2009 Published by Elsevier Inc.

a patient from a previously chronic stable state. Properly framed, these insights provide the practitioner with the necessary skills to identify and manage heart failure, with the ultimate goal of improving care. This article addresses the utility of signs and symptoms and daily weight monitoring in the assessment and management of patients who have heart failure.

DIAGNOSTIC SIGNIFICANCE OF SIGNS AND SYMPTOMS IN HEART FAILURE

A broad range of symptoms, signs, and abnormalities in vital signs, with varying sensitivities and specificities, has been identified in patients who have heart failure (**Box 1**). Symptoms often are related to congestion (eg, dyspnea and abdominal discomfort) or low output (fatigue). Likewise,

---

Box 1
Important findings in chronic heart failure
Symptoms
Dyspnea (rest, exertional, paroxysmal nocturnal dyspnea, orthopnea)
Fatigue
Coughing or wheezing
Chest pain
Palpitations
Anorexia
Weight gain or loss
Depression
Insomnia
Syncope
Transient neurologic symptoms
Signs
Elevated jugular venous pulse
Third heart sound (S3 gallop)
Rales
Dependent edema
Cool extremities
Enlarged point of maximal impulse
Right ventricular lift
Hepatomegaly
Vital sign abnormalities
Hypertension > hypotension
Pulsus alternans
Abnormal Valsalva response
Narrow pulse pressure

---

physical examination findings commonly are related to evidence of congestion (jugular venous distention, pulmonary rales, hepatomegaly, edema) or low cardiac output (cool extremities). Bedside assessment of the vital signs has been useful in the characterization of heart failure, with a focus on heart rate and measurement of blood pressure at rest, under orthostatic conditions, or with the Valsalva maneuver.

ORIGIN OF HEART FAILURE SYMPTOMS

A traditional understanding of the symptoms of chronic heart failure is that its two most common symptoms, fatigue and dyspnea, are the results of distinct mechanisms.[9] Fatigue is attributed to peripheral hypoperfusion that is relayed to the brain via signals from the skeletal muscle, whereas dyspnea is attributed to elevated left ventricular filling pressure. The latter leads to decreased lung compliance and increased airway resistance, increased ventilation–perfusion mismatch caused by increased dead space ventilation, and perhaps increased alveolar wall and blood vessel C-fiber responsiveness to interstitial congestion.[10] More recent data, however, suggest that dyspnea and fatigue may be "two sides of the same coin." Specifically, alterations in peripheral factors, including skeletal muscle fiber profile and metabolism, may contribute to both symptoms, because the hemodynamic profiles of patients reporting fatigue are not significantly different from those reporting dyspnea.[11]

SIGNS AND SYMPTOMS IN DECOMPENSATED HEART FAILURE

Recently, the prevalence of common symptoms and signs in the setting of hospital admission for heart failure decompensation has been reported in large registries such as the Acute Decompensated Heart Failure National Registry (ADHERE), the EuroHeart Failure survey (EURO HF), and the Organized Program to Initiate Lifesaving Treatment in Hospitalized Patients with Heart Failure (OPTIMIZE-HF). Other insights come from large clinical trials in decompensated heart failure, such as Evaluation Study of Congestive Heart Failure and Pulmonary Artery Catheter Effectiveness (ESCAPE) and Efficacy of Vasopressin Antagonism in Heart Failure: Outcome Study with Tolvaptan (EVEREST), and from the accumulated data of smaller trials reporting signs and symptoms.[12] Finally, other registries such as the Epidemiologia da Insuficiencia Cardíaca e Aprendizagem (EPICA) registry have provided similar data from the ambulatory setting.

Dyspnea is the most common symptom reported by patients presenting to the hospital with decompensated heart failure. In ADHERE and OPTIMIZE-HF, approximately 90% of patients reported some dyspnea with approximately one third to one half of patients reporting the presence of dyspnea at rest.[13] Older patients who have decompensated heart failure are less likely to report exertional dyspnea and are more likely to report dyspnea at rest,[14] perhaps because of age or comorbidity leading to functional impairment. The diagnostic utility of dyspnea in this setting is limited by its lack of specificity, vague formal definition, and complex and incompletely understood pathophysiology. Subclassification of dyspnea into dyspnea at rest, immediate dyspnea on light exertion, orthopnea, and paroxysmal nocturnal dyspnea may enhance specificity for elevated filling pressures. In ambulatory patients who had heart failure in the Digitalis Investigation Group trial, 95% of participants reported exertional dyspnea, and 25% reported dyspnea at rest.[15] An analysis of the EPICA registry identified the descriptors dyspnea at rest, orthopnea, and prior paroxysmal nocturnal dyspnea as having high specificity (> 99%) for heart failure.[16] A simple report of dyspnea on any exertion was much less sensitive and specific, although its utility was improved by using specific questions about dyspnea on "normal walking" (specificity, 98%) and "after 90 m at a normal pace" (specificity, 96%). Recently a standardized, scaled approach to the classification of dyspnea in clinical trials has been proposed.[17]

Chest pain is another important symptom in patients who have heart failure. In the Randomized Evaluation of Strategies for Left Ventricular Dysfunction (RESOLVD) study, myocardial ischemia was the precipitant of hospitalization in 12% of cases,[18] and in one emergency department series the incidence of acute coronary syndrome in patients who had chronic heart failure presenting with chest pain was 32%.[19] The presence of chest pain in patients who have heart failure may alert physicians of the need to assess for ischemia. When chest pain is unlikely to be related to fixed epicardial coronary artery stenoses leading to demand ischemia, alternative causes such as myocarditis, pulmonary embolism, and pulmonary hypertension should be considered.

Fatigue is another important symptom to assess in patients who have heart failure, although its reported prevalence in acute decompensated heart failure is surprisingly low in recent registries: 31% in ADHERE[20] and 23% in OPTIMIZE-HF.[13] This low prevalence, however, may represent underreporting in the face of more alarming acute symptoms. Fatigue can be one of the most frustrating and disabling complaints for patients who have heart failure, and it has been linked to other psychologic factors. Comorbid depression is associated with an increased reporting of fatigue and dyspnea[21] and a type D or "distressed" personality type is associated with an increased perception of generalized fatigue in heart failure.[22]

Awareness of the symptoms of clinical depression is important in treating heart failure. Depression is associated with an increased development of heart failure in patients at risk[23] and is associated with an increased likelihood of rehospitalization or death in patients who have a diagnosis of heart failure.[24,25] Severe or worsening heart failure would be expected to generate symptoms of depression, but even after controlling for the severity of heart failure the presence of clinically significant symptoms of depression was associated with a hazard ratio of 1.56 (95% confidence interval [CI], 1.07–2.29) for a composite end point of death or cardiovascular rehospitalization.[26] An even stronger association existed for the use of antidepressant medication and this composite end point, with a hazard ratio of 1.75 (95% CI, 1.14–2.68). Given that these hazard ratios are similar to those associated with traditionally recognized physiologic parameters such as ejection fraction, the relationship between depression and heart failure will be an important focus of clinical practice and research in the future.

Patients or caretakers frequently report cognitive and sleep disturbances. Chronic heart failure is associated with increased cognitive impairment;[27,28] purported mechanisms include cerebral hypoperfusion, hypercoagulability, and cerebral vascular remodeling. Disordered breathing in sleep has been noted in patients who have heart failure; in these patients the prevalence of obstructive sleep apnea is 11% to 37%, and the prevalence of central sleep apnea is 33% to 40%.[29,30] Although obstructive sleep apnea is regarded more as a comorbidity tracking with heart failure, central sleep apnea is thought to be a symptom of heart failure and is independently associated with an increased mortality.[31] Although a recent trial of continuous positive airway pressure in patients who had heart failure did not show overall improved survival,[32] subsequent analysis shows potential benefit in patients who have effective suppression of central sleep apnea.[33]

PHYSICAL EXAMINATION AND HEART FAILURE

The most useful physical examination sign for assessing left ventricular filling pressures in a patient who has heart failure is the jugular venous pressure (JVP). Although the JVP directly represents right-sided filling pressure, the right atrial pressure often mirrors left-sided filling pressures in patients who have chronic heart failure.[34] For example, in a series of 1000 patients referred for cardiac transplantation, the right atrial pressure, dichotomized at more than 10 mm Hg, and the pulmonary capillary wedge pressure (PCWP), dichotomized at more than 22 mm Hg, were concordant (ie, both were elevated, or neither was elevated) in 80% of cases.[34] Hepatojugular reflux, as assessed by an increase of the JVP induced by 10 seconds of continuous pressure on the abdomen, may enhance the sensitivity of an examination of the jugular venous pulse. A positive hepatojugular reflux, in the absence of isolated right ventricular dysfunction, reliably predicts a PCWP greater than 15 mm Hg.[35]

There are several practical considerations in examining the jugular venous pulse (**Box 2**). First, because the internal JVP is not known before the examination, it is important to examine the patient in the sitting position at 90°, because highly elevated JVP may be difficult to appreciate if the top of the column of pulsation is too far cephalad. Second, both sides of the neck should be examined, because anatomic variations may allow visualization on one side only. Third, the external jugular veins also should be examined; phasic changes in pulsation associated with respiration may indicate that the external jugular veins are an acceptable indicator of central venous pressures. The utility of the external jugular veins for estimating central venous pressure has been

reported recently.[36] Finally, compression of the veins inferior to a noted pulsation often is required to differentiate the compressible venous pulsation from the noncompressible carotid arterial pulsation.

Cardiac auscultation is another important focus of the physical examination in patients who have heart failure. Prominent murmurs may indicate valvular heart disease complicating or causing heart failure. The presence of third heart sound (S3) is a classic and important finding in heart failure with independent prognostic significance.[37] Placing the stethoscope bell over the point of maximal impulse, preferably with the patient in left lateral decubitus position, will increase the likelihood of detecting a third heart sound. It can be difficult to hear an S3, and interobserver variability is significant.[38]

Pulmonary auscultation is another important component of the physical examination in patients who have heart failure because wheezes or rales may be heard in decompensated heart failure. Both ADHERE and OPTIMIZE-HF reported the presence of rales in approximately two thirds of patients.[13] In one study of acute heart failure, cough was noted to be present in 69% of patients.[39] Wheezing may be present in chronic heart failure, with a frequency reported as high as one third in a cohort of elderly emergency-room patients who had heart failure.[40] Purported mechanisms of wheezing include reflex bronchoconstriction with increased methacholine responsiveness[41,42] and decreased airway diameter resulting from mucosal edema and intraluminal fluid. In patients who have advanced chronic heart failure, the airspaces may be clear despite elevated left ventricular filling pressures because of hypertrophied lymphatics, and it has been demonstrated that radiographic evidence of pulmonary congestion can be absent even at high PCWP.[43]

In clinical practice, peripheral edema is one of the signs most likely to cause a physician to consider a diagnosis of heart failure. Edema is relatively common in patients who have decompensated heart failure and was present in two thirds of patients in the ADHERE and OPTIMIZE-HF trials.[13] Peripheral edema, however, represents extravascular rather than intravascular volume and may be present in numerous other conditions including obesity, venous insufficiency, nephrotic syndrome, and cirrhosis. Its specificity as a sign is increased in the presence of elevated JVP[44] and, perhaps because it is so easily appreciated on examination, the severity of edema on admission is one of the variables most predictive of length of hospitalization for heart failure.[45]

Box 2
Tips to assist the clinician in the assessment of the jugular venous pressure

1. Begin with the patient sitting upright at 90°. If no pulsation is visible, lower the patient gradually toward the supine position until a pulsation is seen. If no pulsation is seen whether the patient is upright, supine, or at a reclining angle between upright and supine, it will not be possible to estimate the jugular venous pressure.
2. Examine both sides of the neck.
3. Assess both the internal and external jugular veins. If only the external jugular vein is visible, confirm that there are respirophasic changes in the venous pulsation before using it to estimate right atrial pressure.
4. Compress inferior to an identified pulsation to distinguish the noncompressible arterial pulsation from the compressible venous pulsation.

Low systolic blood pressure, sometimes in the range of 70 mm Hg, may be found in patients who have severely depressed systolic function, even though they are largely asymptomatic. Cool lower extremities may alert the clinician to the possibility of inadequate perfusion and the diagnosis of cardiogenic shock. Overall, cardiogenic shock is an uncommon finding in acute heart failure, with a prevalence of less than 2% in the EURO HF, ADHERE, and OPTIMIZE-HF trials.[13] Indeed, hypertension (systolic blood pressure >140 mm Hg) is far more common, with a prevalence of greater than 40% in a large Italian registry of acute heart failure.[46]

Abnormalities of heart rhythm, rate, and pulse variability also provide useful data in the assessment of heart failure. Thirty percent of the patients in the ADHERE trial had a history of atrial fibrillation,[20] and atrial fibrillation was present on the initial EKG in 20% of patients in the OPTIMIZE-HF trial.[47] It was reported as the cause for 22% of heart failure hospitalizations in the RESOLVD study.[18] The presence of an alternating strong and weak pulse, or mechanical alternans, is highly prevalent in chronic heart failure and is indicative of larger left ventricular volumes and lower ejection fractions.[48] A rising heart rate may portend decompensation, although invasive monitoring data indicate that the heart rate does not tend to rise significantly until the 24 hours preceding hospitalization.[49]

Use of the Valsalva maneuver has been proposed to enhance the detection of heart failure and volume overload. Its utility was reviewed recently by Felker and colleagues.[50] In a healthy individual, blood pressure rises briefly with the onset of strain and then falls below baseline until strain is released, at which time the systolic pressure rises rapidly above baseline once more and then returns back to baseline. In individuals who have elevated left-sided filling pressures, blood pressure rises with strain and remains stably elevated throughout the strain, returning to baseline only with strain release (the "square-wave" response) (Fig. 1). In addition to its relationship with elevated left-sided filling pressures,[51–53] the Valsalva response correlates with levels of circulating natriuretic peptides.[54] From a clinical standpoint, the authors have found the Valsalva response to be very useful if the patient can cooperate with the strain phase, has a constant systolic blood pressure, and is not in atrial fibrillation.

Overall, how well do examination findings correlate with invasive hemodynamic assessments? Invasive hemodynamic measurements of right atrial pressure were compared with history and physical examination–derived physician estimates in

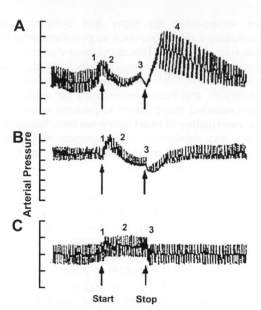

Fig. 1. Blood pressure tracing with Valsalva maneuver in (A) a normal, healthy person, (B) a patient who has mild heart failure with "absent overshoot," (C) and a patient who has severe heart failure with a "square-wave" response. (From Zema MJ, Restivo B, Sos T, et al. Left ventricular dysfunction—bedside Valsalva manoeuvre. Br Heart J 1980;44(5):560–9; with permission.)

patients assigned to the pulmonary artery catheter arm of the ESCAPE trial.[55] Clinician-estimated right atrial pressure of less than 8 mm Hg correlated with measured right atrial pressure of less than 8 mm Hg in 82% of patients, and clinician-estimated right atrial pressure of more than 12 mm Hg correlated with measured right atrial pressure of more than 12 mm Hg in 70% of patients. Overall it seems that physicians can estimate right atrial pressure with reasonable accuracy. Additional components of the history and physical examination were assessed for their ability to predict PCWP. The only history and physical examination findings associated with a PCWP ≥ 30 mm Hg were an estimated right atrial pressure ≥ 12 mm Hg and orthopnea ≥ 2 pillows. In detecting a low cardiac index, only an overall assessment of inadequate perfusion (a "cold" profile) had clinical utility.[55]

PROGNOSTIC SIGNIFICANCE OF SIGNS AND SYMPTOMS IN HEART FAILURE

Acute heart failure syndromes are characterized more by volume overload and hemodynamic congestion than by low cardiac output.[13] Clinically volume overload and hemodynamic congestion are represented by signs and symptoms of increasing congestion, such as peripheral edema, dyspnea, and rales. This development of congestion often goes unrecognized by patients until hospitalization is necessary. Consequently, admission and readmission rates for acute decompensated heart failure in patients who have a known history of heart failure are high. Measurement and monitoring of congestion in chronic heart failure is of great clinical interest for both diagnosis and prognosis. Lucas and colleagues[56] developed a metric for congestion incorporating orthopnea, jugular venous distension, edema, weight gain, and increase from baseline diuretic use in NYHA class IV patients 4 to 6 weeks after hospital discharge. These investigators showed that freedom from congestion was predictive of survival at 2 years, with 87% of patients who had no residual symptoms surviving compared with 67% of patients who had one or two symptoms and 41% of those who had three or more symptoms (**Fig. 2**). Persistence of orthopnea in a clinic population of patients who had heart failure predicted significantly higher 1-year hospitalization rates and failure to improve left ventricular ejection fraction.[57]

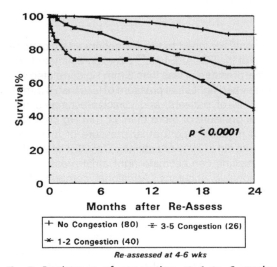

Fig. 2. Persistence of congestion at 4 to 6 weeks following hospital discharge for heart failure decompensation predicts mortality at 2 years. The graph charts the percentage and length of survival in patients in whom no, one or two, or three to five congestion variables were present 4 to 6 weeks after discharge. The variables were orthopnea, JVD, a weight gain of more than 2 lb from the previous week, a need to increase diuretic dosage, and edema. (*From* Lucas C, Johnson W, Hamilton MA, et al. Freedom from congestion predicts good survival despite previous class IV symptoms of heart failure. Am Heart J 2000;140:840; with permission.)

Individual symptoms also may have prognostic significance in heart failure. NYHA class II and III patients participating in the Carvedilol or Metoprolol European Trial self-rated symptoms of heart failure using a five-point scale. By univariate analysis, orthopnea, breathlessness, and fatigue each were associated with a significantly increased relative risk for mortality, all-cause hospitalization, and worsening heart failure.[58] Angina was associated with a significantly increased risk for mortality and all-cause hospitalization but not with worsening heart failure. The relative risk for all outcomes was greatest with orthopnea and least for angina. With multivariate analysis, however, only breathlessness remained a significant predictor of mortality or all-cause hospitalization.

The authors previously assessed the prognostic utility of jugular venous distention and the third heart sound in patients who had heart failure. In a univariate post hoc analysis of the Studies in Left Ventricular Dysfunction trial, JVP and S3 were found to be predictive of subsequent hospitalization for heart failure and of all-cause mortality. In a multivariate model, both were associated with a significantly increased risk of hospitalization for heart failure, death from pump failure, or the composite end point of death or heart failure hospitalization independently of traditional markers of disease severity including NYHA class. The presence of either JVP, S3, or both was associated with all-cause mortality as well (**Fig. 3**).[37] Others also have demonstrated the prognostic utility of S3.[59]

Altered vital signs also convey prognostic significance in heart failure. A recent analysis of beta-blocker trials in heart failure showed a close relationship between the all-cause annualized mortality rate and heart rate on therapy (adjusted $R^2 = 0.51$; $P = .004$) and a strong correlation between a change in heart rate and a change in left ventricular ejection fraction.[60] Systolic blood pressure below 100 mm Hg was reported to be associated with an increased mortality in the N-terminal pro-B-type natriuretic peptide (NT-proBNP) substudy of the Carvedilol Prospective Randomized Cumulative Survival trial (relative risk, 4.13; 95% CI, 2.11–7.70), nearly double the risk found for a NT-proBNP above the mean.[61] For each 10–mm Hg decrease in the pretreatment systolic blood pressure, the risk of death was increased by 18%.[62] Low pulse pressure (the difference between the systolic and diastolic blood pressure) portends a 2.5 times increased risk of death in patients who have decompensated heart failure[63] and is thought to be a marker of low cardiac output.[44]

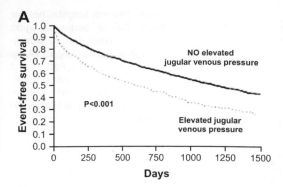

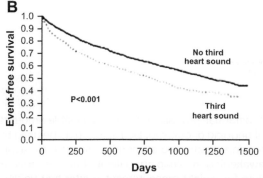

Fig. 3. (*A*) Elevated JVP and (*B*) the presence of S3 confer negative prognosis. (*From* Drazner MH, Rame JE, Stevenson LW, et al. Prognostic importance of elevated jugular venous pressure and a third heart sound in patients with heart failure. N Engl J Med 2001;345:574; with permission.)

DAILY WEIGHT MONITORING IN THE AMBULATORY SETTING

Guidelines for the hospital discharge of patients who have heart failure include the education of patients in the monitoring of daily weights.[64] The utility of monitoring daily weights assumes that a weight increase will precede the development of symptoms during an acute decompensation of heart failure and that an intervention can be implemented that will prevent an adverse event from the decompensation (such as hospitalization).

Patients need to be instructed on how to measure daily weights. Only 11% (range, 2%–20%; $P = .001$) of patients admitted for heart failure in a 1994–1995 survey of University Health System Consortium hospitals received instructions in daily weight monitoring at home.[65] A 2005 survey of care for African American patients at a university teaching hospital showed that only 9% were told to monitor their weight daily.[66] Previous data have shown that cardiologists are more likely than noncardiologists to provide education regarding daily weight monitoring.[67] The Joint Commission on Accreditation of Health

care Organizations now bundles weight-monitoring education with several other discharge instructions in its core performance measure HF-1, one of four core performance measures for heart failure admissions. Not surprisingly, from the third quarter of 2002 to the fourth quarter of 2003, compliance increased significantly from a level of 28% to 55.6%. HF-1, however, is the least conformed to of the core measures.[68]

It is interesting to assess the relationship between weight gain and the state of decompensated heart failure. A study of patients who had NYHA class I to IV heart failure showed little day-to-day correlation between answers on daily symptom questionnaires and self-recorded daily weights,[69] and other small studies demonstrated only a modest incidence (25%–40%) of self-reported weight gain in the weeks preceding admission for decompensated heart failure.[39,70] In contrast, in a case-control trial of patients who had NYHA class III heart failure undergoing telephonically transmitted measurements of daily weights, Chaudhry and colleagues[71] found that hospitalization for heart failure was associated with a mean daily increase in body weight for 1 week before hospitalization for heart failure (**Fig. 4**). Another small trial of patients recently hospitalized for NYHA class IV heart failure found any weight gain to be insensitive for decompensation, but a weight gain greater than 2 kg or a weight gain of 2% over 2 to 3 days (which is the European standard for discharge education of patients) was found to be highly specific for heart failure decompensation.[72] In brief, although weight gain may not always occur before hospitalization, a moderate or persistent weight gain seems to be a useful intermediate-range marker for impending hospitalization and is useful for monitoring.

In the Weight Monitoring in Heart Failure (WHARF) trial, NYHA class III and IV patients who had depressed left ventricular systolic function were assigned randomly to conventional therapy or to telephonically transmitted data monitoring that included daily weight measurements and questions regarding heart failure symptoms. Nurses reported concerning data to physicians and relayed changes in the treatment plan to the patients. There was no statistically significant difference in medication use between the groups at 6 months. Although there was no reduction in the primary end point of 6-month rehospitalization, there was a statistically significant 56% reduction in the secondary end point of mortality at 6 months.[73] This difference in survival disappeared within 6 months after the withdrawal of the intervention.[74] Although symptom reporting was

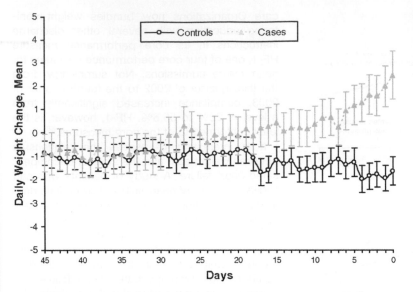

Fig. 4. Patients hospitalized for heart failure begin to gain weight 1 week before admission. (*From* Chaudhry SI, Wang Y, Concato J, et al. Patterns of weight change preceding hospitalization for heart failure. Circulation 2007;116:1549: with permission.)

a component of the WHARF intervention, the investigators concluded that electronic daily weight monitoring may reduce mortality and warrants further study. Subsequently, the Randomized Trial of Telephone Intervention in Chronic Heart Failure trial randomly assigned predominantly NYHA class II and III patients who had systolic dysfunction to a multidisciplinary nurse telephone monitoring program that included patient self-measurement of daily weight. In this trial, there was a significant improvement in the main end point of all-cause mortality or hospital admission for heart failure driven primarily by a reduction in hospitalizations for heart failure.[75]

DAILY WEIGHTS IN THE HOSPITAL

In patients hospitalized for decompensated heart failure, the Heart Failure Society of America guidelines recommend weights be measured daily, along with close monitoring of inputs and outputs. Daily weights in the hospital, considered with input and output measurements, are a useful metric to determine the efficacy of diuretic therapy. In a review of practitioners at Northwestern Memorial Hospital, cardiologists were more likely than non-cardiologists to monitor daily weights.[67] As in the ambulatory setting, however, overall performance in obtaining daily weights was poor. In Canada, daily weights in the hospital were obtained only approximately 20% of the time;[76] data from the United States are lacking.

The authors have noted several practical considerations in the measurement of daily weights. Patients may be weighed either by bed scale or by standing scale in the hospital; inconsistencies in measurement between the two may be

substantial, probably because of variable amounts of bedding or clothing. Bed scales may be used by nursing staff before morning rounds to avoid awakening a sleeping patient, but the optimal time for weight measurement is after first voiding in the morning. The most effective strategy seems to be use of the same standing scale each morning, after voiding, before breakfast, and with the patient wearing the same amount of clothes (eg, undergarments only), a process that requires considerable coordination of planning in the hospital setting.

The amount of weight loss during a hospitalization for decompensated heart failure and the relationship of the weight loss to subsequent outcome is an area of growing interest. In the ADHERE experience, a substantial fraction of patients hospitalized for decompensated heart failure either lost less than 5 lb of weight or gained weight during the hospitalization.[77] In the ESCAPE trial, weight was measured at randomization and at discharge. Median in-hospital weight loss was 2.8 kg (interquartile range, 0.7–6.1 kg), with 17% of patients either gaining weight or losing no weight.[78] A smaller New Zealand study of mostly NYHA class IV patients hospitalized for heart failure showed similar results, with a mean weight loss of 2.8 kg (95% CI, 2.04–31.6).[46] In the ESCAPE trial, significant predictors of weight loss included duration of hospitalization, B-type natriuretic peptide level, and baseline weight. The reciprocal relationship between length of hospitalization and weight loss was demonstrated in the New Zealand study, and change in weight was an independent predictor of a hospital stay of 10 days or greater. The most significant variable affecting length of stay in the New Zealand study was the number of days of treatment with intravenous diuretic, which accounted for 55% of the variance. The relationship between the number of days of treatment with intravenous diuretics and weight loss was not reported in the ESCAPE trial, although there was a minimal association between the maximal diuretic dose and the weight loss achieved ($R^2 = 0.030$) that was insignificant after adjustments for other factors.[78]

The EVEREST trial looked at the short- and long-term benefits of adding tolvaptan, a vasopressin receptor antagonist, to therapy in patients hospitalized for decompensated heart failure who had systolic dysfunction and NYHA class III/IV symptoms.[79] There was a significantly greater loss in body weight at day 1 and at day 7 or discharge for patients in the tolvaptan arm, and this weight loss was associated with some improvements in dyspnea at day 1 and in edema at day 7. After 8 weeks of follow-up, there was no longer a significant difference in weight between the two treatment groups. Further, at day 7 or at discharge, there was no significant difference in patient-assessed global clinical status, and there was no difference in the study primary and secondary end points of all-cause mortality and cardiovascular mortality/hospitalization for heart failure.[80,81]

Although congestion is the predominant cause of hospitalization in patients who have heart failure, the average amount of weight loss achieved by diuresis during the hospitalization seems surprisingly small. There are, however, few data available to suggest that greater weight loss in the hospital would translate into improved outcomes. Further, escalated diuretic doses may be associated with adverse outcomes. Further study is needed to define the optimal in-hospital treatment strategy of patients who have decompensated heart failure.

SUMMARY

The history and physical examination yield immediate and useful information for the diagnosis and management of congestive heart failure. Orthopnea and paroxysmal nocturnal dyspnea are the symptoms most suggestive of heart failure as the cause of dyspnea, and the finding of an elevated jugular venous pulse on physical examination reliably suggests the presence of elevated right atrial pressures, the latter often correlating with elevated left-sided filling pressures. Elevated JVP, S3 gallop, low pulse pressure, and low systolic blood pressure all portend worsened clinical outcomes, as does the overall persistence of symptoms of congestion, particularly orthopnea. Relief of congestion and maintaining freedom from congestion are essential goals of heart failure therapy, and attention is being focused on disease monitoring as a way of anticipating a need for therapeutic intervention. Although measurement of daily weight is critical in the management of heart failure, methods of how best to incorporate this strategy, both in the hospital and in the outpatient setting, need further study. Despite advances in technology, the history and physical examination with a focus on the findings described in this article remain essential for the appropriate assessment and care of patients who have heart failure.

REFERENCES

1. Rosamond W, Flegal K, Furie K, et al. Heart disease and stroke statistics—2008 update: a report from the American Heart Association Statistics Committee and Stroke Statistics Subcommittee. Circulation 2008;117:e25–146.
2. Roger VL, Weston SA, Redfield MM, et al. Trends in heart failure incidence and survival in a community-based population. JAMA 2004;292:344–50.
3. Stewart S, MacIntyre K, Capewell S, et al. Heart failure and the aging population: an increasing burden in the 21st century? Heart 2003;89:49–53.
4. Mangione S, Nieman LZ, Gracely E, et al. The teaching and practice of cardiac auscultation during internal medicine and cardiology training. A nationwide survey. Ann Intern Med 1993;119:47–54.
5. Mangione S, Peitzman SJ, Gracely E, et al. Creation and assessment of a structured review course in physical diagnosis for medical residents. J Gen Intern Med 1994;9:213–8.
6. Laukkanen A, Ikaheimo M, Luukinen H. Practices of clinical examination of heart failure patients in primary health care. Cent Eur J Public Health 2006;14:86–9.
7. Favaloro R. A revival of Paul Dudley White: an overview of present medical practice and of our society. Circulation 1999;99:1525–37.
8. Zoneraich S, Spodick DH. Bedside science reduces laboratory art. Appropriate use of physical findings to reduce reliance on sophisticated and expensive methods. Circulation 1995;91:2089–92.
9. Drexler H, Coats AJ. Explaining fatigue in congestive heart failure. Annu Rev Med 1996;47:241–56.
10. Manning HL, Mahler DA. Pathophysiology of dyspnea. Monaldi Arch Chest Dis 2001;56:325–30.
11. Witte KK, Clark AL. Cycle exercise causes a lower ventilatory response to exercise in chronic heart failure. Heart 2005;91:225–6.
12. Wang CS, FitzGerald JM, Schulzer M, et al. Does this dyspneic patient in the emergency department have congestive heart failure? JAMA 2005;294:1944–56.
13. Gheorghiade M, Filippatos G, De Luca L, et al. Congestion in acute heart failure syndromes: an

essential target of evaluation and treatment. Am J Med 2006;119:S3–10.

14. Ahmed A, Allman RM, Kiefe CI, et al. Association of consultation between generalists and cardiologists with quality and outcomes of heart failure care. Am Heart J 2003;145:1086–93.

15. Ahmed A. Association of diastolic dysfunction and outcomes in ambulatory older adults with chronic heart failure. J Gerontol A Biol Sci Med Sci 2005;60:1339–44.

16. Fonseca C, Morais H, Mota T, et al. The diagnosis of heart failure in primary care: value of symptoms and signs. Eur J Heart Fail 2004;6:795–800.

17. Pang PS, Cleland JG, Teerlink JR, et al. A proposal to standardize dyspnoea measurement in clinical trials of acute heart failure syndromes: the need for a uniform approach. Eur Heart J 2008;29:816–24.

18. Tsuyuki RT, McKelvie RS, Arnold JM, et al. Acute precipitants of congestive heart failure exacerbations. Arch Intern Med 2001;161:2337–42.

19. Lettman NA, Sites FD, Shofer FS, et al. Congestive heart failure patients with chest pain: incidence and predictors of acute coronary syndrome. Acad Emerg Med 2002;9:903–9.

20. Fonarow GC, Heywood JT, Heidenreich PA, et al. Temporal trends in clinical characteristics, treatments, and outcomes for heart failure hospitalizations, 2002 to 2004: findings from Acute Decompensated Heart Failure National Registry (ADHERE). Am Heart J 2007;153:1021–8.

21. Sullivan M, Levy WC, Russo JE, et al. Depression and health status in patients with advanced heart failure: a prospective study in tertiary care. J Card Fail 2004;10:390–6.

22. Smith OR, Michielsen HJ, Pelle AJ, et al. Symptoms of fatigue in chronic heart failure patients: clinical and psychological predictors. Eur J Heart Fail 2007;9:922–7.

23. Abramson J, Berger A, Krumholz HM, et al. Depression and risk of heart failure among older persons with isolated systolic hypertension. Arch Intern Med 2001;161:1725–30.

24. Jiang W, Alexander J, Christopher E, et al. Relationship of depression to increased risk of mortality and rehospitalization in patients with congestive heart failure. Arch Intern Med 2001;161:1849–56.

25. Vaccarino V, Kasl SV, Abramson J, et al. Depressive symptoms and risk of functional decline and death in patients with heart failure. J Am Coll Cardiol 2001;38:199–205.

26. Sherwood A, Blumenthal JA, Trivedi R, et al. Relationship of depression to death or hospitalization in patients with heart failure. Arch Intern Med 2007;167:367–73.

27. Cacciatore F, Abete P, Ferrara N, et al. Congestive heart failure and cognitive impairment in an older population. Osservatorio Geriatrico Campano Study Group. J Am Geriatr Soc 1998;46:1343–8.

28. Taylor J, Stott DJ. Chronic heart failure and cognitive impairment: co-existence of conditions or true association? Eur J Heart Fail 2002;4:7–9.

29. Javaheri S, Parker TJ, Liming JD, et al. Sleep apnea in 81 ambulatory male patients with stable heart failure. Types and their prevalences, consequences, and presentations. Circulation 1998;97:2154–9.

30. Sin DD, Fitzgerald F, Parker JD, et al. Risk factors for central and obstructive sleep apnea in 450 men and women with congestive heart failure. Am J Respir Crit Care Med 1999;160:1101–6.

31. Lanfranchi PA, Braghiroli A, Bosimini E, et al. Prognostic value of nocturnal Cheyne-Stokes respiration in chronic heart failure. Circulation 1999;99:1435–40.

32. Bradley TD, Logan AG, Kimoff RJ, et al. Continuous positive airway pressure for central sleep apnea and heart failure. N Engl J Med 2005;353:2025–33.

33. Arzt M, Floras JS, Logan AG, et al. Suppression of central sleep apnea by continuous positive airway pressure and transplant-free survival in heart failure: a post hoc analysis of the Canadian Continuous Positive Airway Pressure for Patients with Central Sleep Apnea and Heart Failure trial (CANPAP). Circulation 2007;115:3173–80.

34. Drazner MH, Hamilton MA, Fonarow G, et al. Relationship between right and left-sided filling pressures in 1000 patients with advanced heart failure. J Heart Lung Transplant 1999;18:1126–32.

35. Ewy GA. The abdominojugular test: technique and hemodynamic correlates. Ann Intern Med 1988;109:456–60.

36. Vinayak AG, Levitt J, Gehlbach B, et al. Usefulness of the external jugular vein examination in detecting abnormal central venous pressure in critically ill patients. Arch Intern Med 2006;166:2132–7.

37. Drazner MH, Rame JE, Stevenson LW, et al. Prognostic importance of elevated jugular venous pressure and a third heart sound in patients with heart failure. N Engl J Med 2001;345:574–81.

38. Lok CE, Morgan CD, Ranganathan N. The accuracy and interobserver agreement in detecting the 'gallop sounds' by cardiac auscultation. Chest 1998;114:1283–8.

39. Schiff GD, Fung S, Speroff T, et al. Decompensated heart failure: symptoms, patterns of onset, and contributing factors. Am J Med 2003;114:625–30.

40. Jorge S, Becquemin MH, Delerme S, et al. Cardiac asthma in elderly patients: incidence, clinical presentation and outcome. BMC Cardiovasc Disord 2007;7:16.

41. Cabanes LR, Weber SN, Matran R, et al. Bronchial hyperresponsiveness to methacholine in patients with impaired left ventricular function. N Engl J Med 1989;320:1317–22.

42. Moore DP, Weston A, Hughes JM, et al. Bronchial hyperresponsiveness in heart failure. N Engl J Med 1993;328:1424–5.

43. Mahdyoon H, Klein R, Eyler W, et al. Radiographic pulmonary congestion in end-stage congestive heart failure. Am J Cardiol 1989;63:625–7.

44. Stevenson LW, Perloff JK. The limited reliability of physical signs for estimating hemodynamics in chronic heart failure. JAMA 1989;261:884–8.

45. Wright SP, Verouhis D, Gamble G, et al. Factors influencing the length of hospital stay of patients with heart failure. Eur J Heart Fail 2003;5:201–9.

46. Tavazzi L, Maggioni AP, Lucci D, et al. Nationwide survey on acute heart failure in cardiology ward services in Italy. Eur Heart J 2006;27:1207–15.

47. Yancy CW, Lopatin M, Stevenson LW, et al. Clinical presentation, management, and in-hospital outcomes of patients admitted with acute decompensated heart failure with preserved systolic function: a report from the Acute Decompensated Heart Failure National Registry (ADHERE) database. J Am Coll Cardiol 2006;47:76–84.

48. Kodama M, Kato K, Hirono S, et al. Mechanical alternans in patients with chronic heart failure. J Card Fail 2001;7:138–45.

49. Adamson PB, Magalski A, Braunschweig F, et al. Ongoing right ventricular hemodynamics in heart failure: clinical value of measurements derived from an implantable monitoring system. J Am Coll Cardiol 2003;41:565–71.

50. Felker GM, Cuculich PS, Gheorghiade M. The Valsalva maneuver: a bedside "biomarker" for heart failure. Am J Med 2006;119:117–22.

51. McIntyre KM, Vita JA, Lambrew CT, et al. A noninvasive method of predicting pulmonary-capillary wedge pressure. N Engl J Med 1992;327:1715–20.

52. Givertz MM, Slawsky MT, Moraes DL, et al. Noninvasive determination of pulmonary artery wedge pressure in patients with chronic heart failure. Am J Cardiol 2001;87:1213–5.

53. Sharma GV, Woods PA, Lambrew CT, et al. Evaluation of a noninvasive system for determining left ventricular filling pressure. Arch Intern Med 2002;162:2084–8.

54. Brunner-La Rocca HP, Weilenmann D, Rickli H, et al. Is blood pressure response to the Valsalva maneuver related to neurohormones, exercise capacity, and clinical findings in heart failure? Chest 1999;116:861–7.

55. Drazner MH, Hellkamp AS, Leier CV, et al. Value of clinician assessment of hemodynamics in advanced heart failure: The ESCAPE trial. Circ Heart Fail 2008;1:170–7.

56. Lucas C, Johnson W, Hamilton MA, et al. Freedom from congestion predicts good survival despite previous class IV symptoms of heart failure. Am Heart J 2000;140:840–7.

57. Beck da Silva L, Mielniczuk L, Laberge M, et al. Persistent orthopnea and the prognosis of patients in the heart failure clinic. Congest Heart Fail 2004; 10:177–80.

58. Ekman I, Cleland JG, Swedberg K, et al. Symptoms in patients with heart failure are prognostic predictors: insights from COMET. J Card Fail 2005;11:288–92.

59. Acanfora D, Crisci C, Rengo C, et al. Clinical determinants of long-term mortality in elderly patients with heart disease. Arch Gerontol Geriatr 1995;21:233–40.

60. Flannery G, Gehrig-Mills R, Billah B, et al. Analysis of randomized controlled trials on the effect of magnitude of heart rate reduction on clinical outcomes in patients with systolic chronic heart failure receiving beta-blockers. Am J Cardiol 2008;101:865–9.

61. Hartmann F, Packer M, Coats AJ, et al. Prognostic impact of plasma N-terminal pro-brain natriuretic peptide in severe chronic congestive heart failure: a substudy of the Carvedilol Prospective Randomized Cumulative Survival (COPERNICUS) trial. Circulation 2004;110:1780–6.

62. Rouleau JL, Roecker EB, Tendera M, et al. Influence of pretreatment systolic blood pressure on the effect of carvedilol in patients with severe chronic heart failure: the Carvedilol Prospective Randomized Cumulative Survival (COPERNICUS) study. J Am Coll Cardiol 2004;43:1423–9.

63. Aronson D, Burger AJ. Relation between pulse pressure and survival in patients with decompensated heart failure. Am J Cardiol 2004;93:785–8.

64. Bonow RO, Bennett S, Casey DE Jr, et al. ACC/AHA clinical performance measures for adults with chronic heart failure: a report of the American College Of Cardiology/American Heart Association Task Force on Performance Measures (Writing Committee to Develop Heart Failure Clinical Performance Measures) endorsed by the Heart Failure Society of America. J Am Coll Cardiol 2005;46: 1144–78.

65. Nohria A, Chen YT, Morton DJ, et al. Quality of care for patients hospitalized with heart failure at academic medical centers. Am Heart J 1999;137:1028–34.

66. Ilksoy N, Moore RH, Easley K, et al. Quality of care in African-American patients admitted for congestive heart failure at a university teaching hospital. Am J Cardiol 2006;97:690–3.

67. Patel JA, Fotis MA. Comparison of treatment of patients with congestive heart failure by cardiologists versus noncardiologists. Am J Health Syst Pharm 2005;62:168–72.

68. Fonarow GC, Yancy CW, Heywood JT. Adherence to heart failure quality-of-care indicators in US hospitals: analysis of the ADHERE registry. Arch Intern Med 2005;165:1469–77.

69. Webel AR, Frazier SK, Moser DK, et al. Daily variability in dyspnea, edema and body weight in heart failure patients. Eur J Cardiovasc Nurs 2007;6:60–5.

70. Jurgens CY. Somatic awareness, uncertainty, and delay in care-seeking in acute heart failure. Res Nurs Health 2006;29:74–86.

71. Chaudhry SI, Wang Y, Concato J, et al. Patterns of weight change preceding hospitalization for heart failure. Circulation 2007;116:1549–54.

72. Lewin J, Ledwidge M, O'Loughlin C, et al. Clinical deterioration in established heart failure: what is the value of BNP and weight gain in aiding diagnosis? Eur J Heart Fail 2005;7:953–7.

73. Goldberg LR, Piette JD, Walsh MN, et al. Randomized trial of a daily electronic home monitoring system in patients with advanced heart failure: the Weight Monitoring in Heart Failure (WHARF) trial. Am Heart J 2003;146:705–12.

74. Niya AJ, David SF, John DP, et al. Withdrawal of a technology-based daily weight monitoring system in patients with advanced heart failure eliminates mortality benefit. J Card Fail 2007;13: S179.

75. GESICA. Randomised trial of telephone intervention in chronic heart failure: DIAL trial. BMJ 2005;331: 425.

76. Tu J DL, Lee D, Ko D, et al. Quality of cardiac care in Ontario: EFFECT study phase I. Report 2. Toronto (Canada): Institute for Clinical Evaluative Sciences; 2006.

77. Fonarow GC. The Acute Decompensated Heart Failure National Registry (ADHERE): opportunities to improve care of patients hospitalized with acute decompensated heart failure. Rev Cardiovasc Med 2003;4(Suppl 7):S21–30.

78. Hasselblad V, Gattis Stough W, Shah MR, et al. Relation between dose of loop diuretics and outcomes in a heart failure population: results of the ESCAPE trial. Eur J Heart Fail 2007;9:1064–9.

79. Gheorghiade M, Orlandi C, Burnett JC, et al. Rationale and design of the multicenter, randomized, double-blind, placebo-controlled study to evaluate the efficacy of vasopressin antagonism in heart failure: outcome study with tolvaptan (EVEREST). J Card Fail 2005;11:260–9.

80. Konstam MA, Gheorghiade M, Burnett JC Jr, et al. Effects of oral tolvaptan in patients hospitalized for worsening heart failure: the EVEREST outcome trial. JAMA 2007;297:1319–31.

81. Gheorghiade M, Konstam MA, Burnett JC Jr, et al. Short-term clinical effects of tolvaptan, an oral vasopressin antagonist, in patients hospitalized for heart failure: the EVEREST clinical status trials. JAMA 2007;297:1332–43.

Transthoracic Impedance Cardiography: A Noninvasive Method of Hemodynamic Assessment

Melike Bayram, MD[a],*, Clyde W. Yancy, MD[b]

KEYWORDS

- Thoracic impedance • Impedance cardiography
- Hemodynamic • Noninvasive

The heart failure population is rapidly growing with more than 5 million patients being diagnosed. Each year there are more than 1 million hospitalizations for decompensated heart failure.[1] Although a comprehensive definition of acute decompensated heart failure [ADHF] has yet to be clearly defined and the precise pathophysiology remains unknown, ADHF can be viewed in part as a hemodynamic disorder characterized by elevated atrial and ventricular pressures and in some patients, a decreased cardiac output is also present. These hemodynamic changes lead to the presenting symptoms of decompensated heart failure with decreased exercise capacity, fatigue, worsening dyspnea, paroxysmal nocturnal dyspnea, orthopnea, abdominal distention, and lower extremity edema. Management of acute decompensation is separate from chronic management of heart failure and includes intravenous diuretics with or without vasodilator agents and occasionally inotropic agents based on presentation of the individual patient. Patients who are congested and have signs of low perfusion or frank hypotension are described as "cold and wet" and may require intravenous inotropic agents to boost their cardiac output and improve organ perfusion. Patients who are congested but do not have any signs of low perfusion are described as "warm and wet" and can be managed by intravenous diuretics in addition to vasodilators (intravenous introglycerine, nitroprusside, or nesiritide) if compelling symptoms are present at rest.

Traditionally, history taking and physical examination skills provide the most value in the hemodynamic assessment but bedside assessments are not always accurate. Studies show that clinicians accurately predict volume and perfusion status only 50% of the time when using clinical skills only.[2–5] One report generated a sensitivity at best of only 58% for clinical signs indicative of elevated pulmonary capillary wedge pressures.[4] A narrow pulse pressure has been associated with a low cardiac index but even that simple sign is not always identified. These shortcomings have led to an effort to measure volume and perfusion status more directly and to use those measurements to inform hemodynamic-guided therapy. Hemodynamics can be determined invasively or noninvasively.

[a] The Ohio State University, Columbus, OH, USA
[b] Baylor University Medical Center, Dallas, TX, USA
* Corresponding author. Division of Cardiovascular Medicine, The Ohio State University, 473 West 12th Avenue, Suite 200, Columbus, OH 43210-1225.
E-mail address: melike.bayram@osumc.edu (M. Bayram).

Heart Failure Clin 5 (2009) 161–168
doi:10.1016/j.hfc.2008.12.001
1551-7136/08/$ – see front matter. Published by Elsevier Inc.

PULMONARY ARTERY CATHETER–GUIDED THERAPY

Invasive hemodynamics with pulmonary artery catheter placement enables direct measurement of right atrial, right ventricular, pulmonary systolic, and diastolic pressures as well as pulmonary capillary wedge pressure, which estimates left ventricular end diastolic pressure. Cardiac output can also be determined using either the thermodilution method or the Fick method. Besides providing a better understanding of the clinical picture, hemodynamics provides prognostic data. Elevated pulmonary capillary wedge pressure (PCWP)[6] as well as low cardiac index and elevated systemic resistance[7] are poor prognostic indicators and are associated with increased mortality. In terms of management, hemodynamic data prompt and direct the use of intravenous agents such as diuretics and also provide understanding of the perfusion state, hence supporting the decision to add parenteral vasodilatory therapy or inotropic agents. The overarching concern regarding the availability of any hemodynamic data other than blood pressure in the setting of ADHF is "does the information matter?" Despite the apparent usefulness of invasive hemodynamic measurements, data from the recent ESCAPE (Evaluation Study of Congestive Heart Failure and Pulmonary Artery Catheterization Effectiveness) trial do not support use of pulmonary artery catheters (PAC).[8] This study looked at safety and importance of using pulmonary artery catheters in management of decompensated heart failure and did not find any benefit of using PACs when compared with therapy guided by clinical assessment. Addition of PAC to clinical assessment increased anticipated adverse events, mainly infection, but did not improve mortality or re-hospitalization. These findings do not mean that hemodynamic assessment is not important; rather, that the invasive determination of hemodynamic status is not superior to clinical assessment in patients not in overt cardiogenic shock or with some other clear indication for hemodynamic monitoring. The authors concluded that future trials might study noninvasive methods that could be used to better tailor therapy for both survival time and quality of life.

IMPEDANCE CARDIOGRAPHY

Impedance cardiography (ICG) is a noninvasive method based on Ohm's law that determines changes in thoracic fluid content based on changes in the conductivity/resistance to propagation of an electrical impulse across the thorax. The electrical properties of certain tissues (lungs, vessels, bones, skeletal muscle, and extravascular fluid) vary and conduct alternating current (AC) at differing resistances. One standard method uses 8 symmetrically placed electrodes on the chest wall and the neck. Half of these[4] are current and the other half[4] are voltage electrodes. A low intensity alternating current is passed through the current electrodes as the voltage is measured by the voltage electrodes.[9,10] By Ohm's law, voltage is equal to impedance times the current. As the current of constant intensity flows through the chest wall, amplitude of the voltage measured by the voltage electrodes is directly related to the impedance of the chest contents. The entire resistance of the chest, also known as the basic resistance (Z_0), is the sum of the resistances for each component in the chest (lungs, air, vessels, bones, skeletal muscle, and so forth). Impedance varies with the amount of fluid in the body: when the fluid increases, impedance falls and conductivity rises; and when the fluid content decreases, impedance increases and conductivity falls. Resistance also varies with air volume of lungs with inspiration and expiration, and blood volume and velocity in the vasculature during systole and diastole. Changes in resistance secondary to breathing are filtered out electronically.[9,11,12] Changes secondary to outflow of blood are analyzed (ΔZ) in relation to time and surface EKG. Impedance cardiographs are constructed such that a fall in impedance causes an increase in the value on the y-axis. When gated to an electrocardiogram, the difference in resistance to an electrical current between systole and diastole approximates cardiac stroke volume barring any other acute fluid shifts or changes in chest/thorax resistance.

ICG waveforms have been described in detail in a review by Bour and Kellet.[13] The first derivative waveform (ΔZ) has a velocity S wave that corresponds to fluid velocity during systole. Large S wave indicates a high cardiac output. The initial slope of the S wave correlates with contractility. Steeper slope corresponds to better contractility (**Fig. 1**).[13] The second derivative (dZ/dt), which describes fluid acceleration, is a more detailed waveform with several wave points: a, b, c, x, o (see **Fig. 1**). The "a" wave is related to changes in volume during atrial contraction. The "b" wave appears with aortic valve opening. The "c" point ($\Delta Z/\Delta t$) marks the maximum acceleration of blood out of both ventricles. The $\Delta Z/\Delta t$ reflects changes in volume both in the ascending aorta and in the pulmonary trunk. The aorta has several times greater influence on the "c" value than the pulmonary trunk with changes in impedance being caused by the aorta in 80% of the cases.[14,15] The steepness of the slope of ascent between

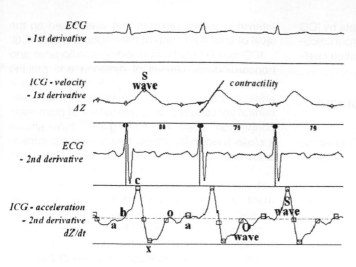

Fig. 1. Impedance cardiography. The slope of the initial part of the S wave correlates with cardiac contractility. The wave's height and width of S wave correlate with the stroke volume. Point "a" correlates with the late diastolic filling; point "b" approximates the opening of aortic valve; point "c" takes place at the maximum acceleration of blood out of the ventricles; point "x" is the point of aortic valve closure; peak of "o" wave corresponds to the peak diastolic flow (E wave on Doppler echocardiography). (*From* Bour J, Kellet J. Impedance cardiography—a rapid and cost-effective screening tool for cardiac disease. Eur J Int Med 2008;19:399-405; with permission.)

b and c points predicts contractility (the steeper the slope the better the contractility). After the "c" wave there is rapid deceleration to the "x" point, which is the point of intrathoracic fluid inversion. The "x" wave roughly corresponds to the aortic valve closure. After the nadir of the "x" point, the waveform returns to baseline and forms the early diastolic waveform "o wave," which is associated with the opening of the mitral valve, and corresponds to the peak of transmitral E wave detected by Doppler echocardiography. The ratio of "o" wave height to S wave height has been shown to have a direct correlation with PCWP; a ratio of 0.5 being equivalent to PCWP of 10 mm Hg.[13,16]

Impedance cardiography directly measures certain parameters, whereas others are calculated. Directly measured parameters include heart rate, thoracic fluid content (1/baseline impedance [/k ohm]), velocity index (first time derivative/baseline impedance [/1000sec]), acceleration index (second time derivative/baseline impedance [/100 second]), pre-ejection period (time from EKG Q wave to aortic valve opening [ms]), and left ventricular ejection time (time from atrioventricular [AV] opening to AV closing [ms]).

Calculated parameters include stroke volume (SV), stroke index, cardiac output (CO), cardiac index (CI), systemic vascular resistance (SVR), systemic vascular resistance index, left cardiac work index, and systolic time ratio.

There are some limitations to the accuracy of ICG measurements. For accurate calculation of stroke volume and cardiac output, it should not be used in patients shorter than 4 feet and taller than 7 feet, and also weighing less than 67 lb or more than 341 lb. Also, extreme tachycardia (HR > 250), severe aortic regurgitation, presence of aortic balloon pump, and severe sepsis interfere

with the accuracy of measurements and ICG should not be used under these circumstances.

STUDIES COMPARING IMPEDANCE CARDIOGRAPHY WITH INVASIVE METHODS

ICG was first advanced in 1940 by Nyboer and colleagues;[17] however, the method has not fully entered clinical practice because it has shown inconsistent performance[18,19] and has not always been deemed well-validated sufficiently to inform clinical decisions. However, within the last 10 years, advances in digital signal processing have enabled ICG to enter clinical practice mainly in assessment of CO.[20] One study[21] showed that the latest generation of ICG algorithm for cardiac output (impedance modulating aortic compliance, aka Z MARC) is superior to previous algorithms.

Verhoeve and colleagues[22] have shown reasonable intraday correlation and expected interday correlation of hemodynamic parameters among stable cardiac rehabilitation patients. This is important for the reproducibility of the measurements. Greenberg and colleagues[11] have also reported reasonable intraday and interday variability of ICG parameters in heart failure patients. Higher variability is expected among heart failure patients because they are more prone to fluid shifts on a day-to-day or even hour-to-hour basis because of the pathophysiology of the disease.

The latest generation of ICG devices has also been compared against traditional invasive methods of measuring CO and CI (by thermodilution [TD] and Fick methods). Van De Water and Miller[21] showed, among post coronary bypass surgery patients, that cardiac outputs calculated by ICG were comparable to cardiac output calculations by thermodilution based on invasive measurements. Other studies also validated the accuracy of cardiac output measurements by ICG by comparing it to Fick or TD cardiac output calculations (**Table 1**). These reported correlation coefficients ranged from 0.73 to 0.93.

CLINICAL USE OF IMPEDANCE CARDIOGRAPHY IN HEART FAILURE

We should be careful including cost data as no cost-effectiveness data have been published regarding the use of ICG in heart failure. For something to be cost effective it must show definitive benefit, which is suggested but not yet evident based on all or the published work. Taler and colleagues[25] used ICG in a study of 104 patients with poorly controlled blood pressure despite being on two or more antihypertensives. Patients were randomized into two groups: one group was treated based on ICG findings and the second group was treated with standard therapy. Proper blood pressure control was achieved 70% more often in the ICG group. Patients in this group had a greater reduction in SVR and were on more

intensive diuretic regimen that was based on the level of total fluid content data obtained from ICG.

ICG can be useful in deciding cardiogenic and noncardiogenic causes of dyspnea and making therapeutic decisions in the acute setting. Impedance cardiography can be used to determine central venous pressures and extent of pulmonary congestion. Ebert and colleagues[26] have shown a close linear relationship between chest impedance and central venous pressures. Data from ED-IMPACT[31] indicate that hemodynamic data obtained by use of ICG led to a change in treatment of 24% of the patients with dyspnea, whereas B type natriuretic peptide (BNP) caused a change in treatment of 11% of similar patients. Springfield and colleagues[32] obtained significant differences in cardiac index (2.2 versus. 3.1, $P < .0001$) and velocity index (32.9 versus. 42.7, $P < .01$) between patients with cardiogenic and noncardiogenic causes of dyspnea. Other studies in the acute setting showed that ICG parameters measured at the emergency department (ED) may predict length of stay.[33] ICG and

Table 1
Validation studies comparing impedance cardiography with invasive methods of cardiac output estimation

Study	Study Size	Comparison Parameters	Correlation Coefficient (R value[a])
Yung et al. (1999)[23]	N = 33 (Pulmonary HTN)	Fick CO – ICG CO TD CO – Fick CO ICG CO – TD CO	0.85 0.89 0.80
Ziegler et al. (1999)[24]	N = 52 (Mechanically ventilated)	ICG CO – TD CO	0.89
Drazner et al. (2002)[27]	N = 59 (Heart failure in cath lab)	ICG CO – Fick CO TD CO – Fick CO ICG CO – TD CO	0.73 0.81 0.76
Sageman et al. (2002)[28]	N = 20 (Post CABG)	ICG CO – TD CO	0.93
Albert et al. (2003)[29]	N = 38 (Heart failure in intensive care unit)	ICG CO – TD CO	0.89
Van De Water and Miller (2003)[21]	N = 53 (Post CABG)	ICG CO - TD CO	0.81
Suttner et al. (2005)[58]	N = 40 (Hemodynamically stable post cardiac surgery) N = 34 (Hemodynamically unstable post cardiac surgery)	ICG CO – TD CO ICG CO– TD CO	0.83 0.79
Scherhag (2005)[30]	N = 20 (CAD) Rest Exercise	ICG CO– TD CO ICG CO– TD CO	0.85 0.92

Abbreviations: CO, cardiac output; ICG, impedance cardiography; TD, theromodilution.
[a] Pearson correlation coefficient.

BNP levels measured at ED also were shown to have 75% prognostic accuracy for readmissions and death within 90 days.[34] This use of ICG to resolve the origin of dyspnea and to augment the diagnostic utility of biomarkers might represent the most reasonable use of ICG for ADHF.

Hemodynamic data obtained by ICG can be used in the diagnosis and treatment of heart failure.[9,25,32,35–37] Numerous studies have reported clinical utility in prospective heart failure treatment.[35–40] Vijayaraghavan and colleagues[36] demonstrated prognostic role of hemodynamic parameters from ICG in patients with chronic heart failure and the strong correlation between these parameters and functional class and quality of life. Recently, the pilot study, PREDICT (Prospective Evaluation and Identification of Decompensation by ICG Test) has demonstrated that when performed at regular intervals in stable patients with heart failure with a recent episode of clinical decompensation, ICG can identify patients at increased near-term risk of recurrent decompensation.[41] The three ICG parameters that were powerful predictors of an event within 14 days when combined into a composite score were velocity index, thoracic fluid content index, and systolic ventricular ejection time. These provocative data need to be prospectively tested in a larger trial, which is ongoing.

Hemodynamic data obtained from ICG can also be used to investigate the influence of medicines on hemodynamic parameters and help make decisions for initiation and up-titration of beta blockers and angiotensinonongen converting enzyme inhibitor therapy.[42,43] In the setting of acute decompensation, assessment of CI, systemic vascular resistance index, thoracic fluid content, and acceleration index (ACI) by impedance cardiography may help determine the need and optimal selection and dosing of intravenous therapy (nesiritide versus. inotropic agents such as milrinone and dobutamine).[37] However, validation studies of ICG versus. invasive hemodynamic monitoring are needed to support the use of ICG in this setting. ICG parameters can also be used in optimizing left ventricular assist device (LVAD) settings and to wean patients off LVAD support in place of parameters obtained invasively.[44]

Impedance cardiography has been used during cardiac pacemaker programming to obtain the optimum atrioventricular settings in DDD pacemakers[45–50] as well as in cardiac resynchronization therapy (CRT).[51–57] Braun and colleagues[54] compared impedance cardiography with Doppler echocardiography for AV interval optimization among 24 patients with New York Heart Association (NYHA) class III-IV heart failure (ejection fraction < 35% and with left bundle branch block [QRS > 150 msec]) within 1 month of receiving resynchronization therapy. AV-interval optimization based on CO calculated by ICG correlated closely with what was obtained based on transaortic flow by Doppler echocardiography.[54] ICG has also been shown as a useful tool in optimization of interventricular (VV) intervals. Heinroth and colleagues[56] studied 46 patients post cardiac resynchronization therapy 3 to 5 days after implantation of the CRT device. They showed that proportion on nonresponders to CRT therapy decreased by 56% following AV and VV optimization based on CO measurements by ICG.

ICG has also been suggested as an adjunct to post–heart transplant myocardial biopsies. Nolert and colleagues[57] showed that a decrease of 20% in ACI obtained by ICG has a sensitivity of 71% and specificity of 100% for graft rejection. This may aid to reduce the number of biopsies. More studies are needed to explore this provocative use of ICG.

SUMMARY

Impedance cardiography technology, along with recent advances in the ICG device, has become a provocative but not yet proven noninvasive alternative to invasive hemodynamic measurements. Validity of ICG measurements has been tested among different populations of patients (see **Table 1**). The results from stroke volume and cardiac output measurements by ICG show reasonably accurate correlation to the values calculated from direct measurements from pulmonary artery catheters. Some studies show that variations between different measurements of thermodilutional (TD) cardiac output (CO) measurements and that between TD CO and ICG CO are similar,[21] which means these methods can be used interchangeably in the right setting. Again, the primary question is which measurement matters for which clinical scenario.

ICG may be a useful adjunct to clinical judgment for heart failure patients. Most institutions continue to use pulmonary artery catheters for direct assessment of hemodynamics because this has been the gold standard, especially among critically ill heart failure patients when critical decisions are being made. The available data would not yet support supplanting invasive hemodynamic assessment in the critical care setting with ICG. ICG may however easily replace repeated pulmonary artery catheter measurements especially in a stable population of heart failure patients where hemodynamic data might inform certain clinical decisions such as in resolution of the origin of dyspnea, CRT optimization, and medication adjustments. Future studies and advances in technology are expected to improve impedance cardiography, thus broadening the clinical applications of this unique technology. Importantly, ongoing research must confirm the precise benefits of this information in order for ICG monitoring to become a standard assessment in heart failure.

REFERENCES

1. Fonarow GC, Adams KF, Abraham WT, et al. Risk stratification for in-hospital mortality in acutely decompensated heart failure: classification and regression tree analysis. JAMA 2005;293:572–80.

2. Speroff T, Connors AF Jr, Dawson NV. Lens model analysis of hemodynamic status in the critically ill. Med Decis Making 1989;9(4):243–52.

3. Eisenberg PR, Jaffe AS, Schuster DP. Clinical evaluation compared to pulmonary artery catheterization in the hemodynamic assessment of critically ill patients. Crit Care Med 1984;12(7):549–53.

4. Stevenson LW, Perloff JK. The limited reliability of physical signs for estimating hemodynamics in chronic heart failure. JAMA 1989;261:884–8.

5. Jonas M, Bruce R, Knight J. Clinical assessment of cardiac output (CO) vs. Lidco indicator kelution (ID) measurement: are clinical estimates of cardiac output and oxygen delivery reliable enough to manage critically ill patients? [abstract]. Crit Care Med 2003;30(12):A68.

6. Fonarow GC, Stevenson LW, Steimle AE, et al. Persistently high left ventricular filling pressures predict mortality despite angiotensin converting enzyme inhibition in advanced heart failure [abstract]. Circulation 1994;90(pt 2):I-488.

7. Huang CM, Young MS, Wei J. Predictors of short term outcome in Chinese patients with ambulatory heart failure for heart transplantation with ejection fraction <25%. Jpn Heart J 2000;41(3):349–69.

8. The ESCAPE Investigators and ESCAPE study Coordinators. Evaluation study of congestive heart failure and pulmonary artery catheterization effectiveness. JAMA 2005;294:1625–33.

9. Strobeck J, Silver M. Beyond the four quadrants: the critical and emerging role of impedance cardiography in heart failure. Congest Heart Fail 2004; 10(Suppl 2):1–6.

10. BioZ ICG monitor user manual. San Diego (CA): CardioDynamics; 2001.

11. Greenberg BH, Hermann DD, Pranulis MF, et al. Reproducibility of impedance cardiography hemodynamic measures in clinically stable heart failure patients. Congest Heart Fail 2000;6(2):19–26, 74–80.

12. Engoren M, Barbee D. Comparison of cardiac output determined by bioimpedance, thermodilution, and the Fick method. Am J Crit Care 2005;14:40–5.

13. Bour J, Kellet J. Impedance cardiography—a rapid and cost-effective screening tool for cardiac disease. Eur J Int Med 2008;19:399–405.

14. Ito H, Yamakoshi K, Yamada A. Physiological and fluid-dynamic investigation of the thoracic impedance plethysmography method for measuring cardiac output: part II. Analysis of thoracic impedance wave by perfusing dog. Med Biol Eng 1976;14:373–8.

15. Thomsen A. Impedance cardiography. Is the output from the right or left ventricle measured? Intensive Care Med 1979;5:206.

16. Woltjer HH, Bogaard HJ, Bronzwaer JGF, et al. Prediction of pulmonary capillary wedge pressure and assessment of stroke volume by noninvasive impedance cardiography. Am Heart J 1997;134: 450–5.

17. Nyboer J, Bagno S, Barnett A, et al. Radiocardiograms: electrical impedance changes in the heart in relation to electrocardiograms and heart sounds. J Clin Invest 1940;2(4):263–70.

18. Belardinelli R, Ciampani N, Costantini C, et al. Comparison of impedance cardiography with thermodilution and direct fick methods for noninvasive measurement of stroke volume and cardiac output during incremental exercise in patients with ischemic cardiomyopathy. Am J Cardiol 1996;77: 1293–301.

19. Marik PE, Penndelton JE, Smith R. A comparison of hemodynamic parameters derived from transthoracic electrical bioimpedance with those parameters obtained by thermodilution and ventricular angiography. Crit Care Med 1997;25(9):1545–50.

20. Linton DM. Advances in noninvasive cardiac output monitoring. Ann Card Anaesth 2002;5:141–8.

21. Van De Water JM, Miller TW. Impedance cardiography: the next vital sign technology? Chest 2003; 123(6):2028–33.

22. Verhoeve PE, Cadwell CA, Tsadok S. Reproducibility of noninvasive bioimpedance measurements of cardiac function [abstract]. J Card Fail 1998; 4(3 Suppl):53.

23. Yung GL, Fletcher CC, Fedullo PF, et al. Noninvasive cardiac index using bioimpedance in comparison to direct fick and thermodilution methods in patients with pulmonary hypertension [abstract]. Chest 1999;116(4):281S.

24. Ziegler D, Grotti L, Krucke G. Comparison of cardiac output measurements by TEB vs. intermittent bolus thermodilution in mechanical ventilated patients [abstract]. Chest 1999;116(4):281S.

25. Taler SJ, Textor SC, Augustine JE. Resistant hypertension: comparing hemodynamic management to specialist care. Hypertension 2002;39:982–8.

26. Ebert TJ, Smith JJ, Barney JA, et al. The use of thoracic impedance for determining thoracic blood

volume changes in man. Aviat Space Environ Med 1986;57:49–53.

27. Drazner M, Thompson B, Rosenberg P, et al. Comparison of impedance cardiography with invasive hemodynamic measurements in patients with heart failure secondary to ischemic or nonischemic cardiomyopathy. Am J Cardiol 2002;89(8):993–5.

28. Sageman WS, Riffenburgh RH, Spiess BD. Equivalence of bioimpedance and thermodilution in measuring cardiac index after cardiac surgery. J Cardiothorac Vasc Anesth 2002;16(1):8–14.

29. Albert N, Hail M, Li J, et al. Equivalence of bioimpedance and TD in measuring CO/CI in patients with advanced, decompensated chronic heart failure hosp. in critical care [abstract]. J Am Coll Cardiol 2003;41(6 Suppl):211A.

30. Scherhag A, Kaden JJ, Kentschke T, et al. Comparison of impedance cardiography and thermodilution-derived measurements of stroke volume and cardiac output at rest and during exercise testing. Cardiovasc Drugs Ther 2005;19:141–7.

31. Peacock WF, Summers RL, Vogel J, et al. Impact of impedance cardiography on diagnosis and therapy of emergent dyspnea: the ED-IMPACT trial. Acad Emerg Med 2006;13:365–71.

32. Springfield CL, Sebat F, Johnson D, et al. Utility of impedance cardiography to determine cardiac vs. noncardiac cause of dyspnea in the emergency department. Congest Heart Fail 2004;10(Suppl 2):14–6.

33. Milzman D, Samaddar R, Napoli A, et al. The predictive value of noninvasive impedance cardiography in determining patient outcome in acute heart failure: a prospective blinded study [abstract]. Ann Emerg Med 2000;36(4):S4–5.

34. Kazanegra R, Barcarse E, Chen A, et al. Plasma levels of B type natriuretic peptide (BNP) and non-invasive cardiac index in diagnosing congestive heart failure in the emergency department [abstract]. J Card Fail 2002;8(Suppl):S84.

35. Silver MA, Cianci P, Brennan S, et al. Evaluation of impedance cardiography as an alternative to pulmonary artery catheterization in critically ill patients. Congest Heart Fail 2004;10(Suppl 2):17–21.

36. Vijayaraghavan K, Crum S, Cherukuri S, et al. Association of impedance cardiography parameters with changes in functional and quality-of-life measures in patients with chronic heart failure. Congest Heart Fail 2004;10(Suppl 2):22–7.

37. Lasater M. Managing inotrope therapy noninvasively. AACN Clin Issues 1999;10:406–13.

38. Rosenberg P, Yancy CW. Noninvasive assessment of hemodynamics: an emphasis on impedance cardiography. Curr Opin Cardiol 2000;15:151–5.

39. Wright RF, Gilbert J. Clinical decision making in patients with congestive heart failure: the role of thoracic electrical bioimpedance. Congest Heart Fail 2000;6(2):81–5.

40. Strobeck JE, Silver MA, Ventura H. Impedance cardiography: noninvasive measurement of cardiac stroke volume and thoracic fluid content. Congest Heart Fail 2000;6(2):56–9.

41. Packer M, Abraham WT, Mehra MR, et al. Utility of impedance cardiography for identification of short-term risk of clinical decompensation in stable patients with chronic heart failure. J Am Coll Cardiol 2006;47:2245–52.

42. Hayes DL, Hayes SN, Hyberger LK, et al. Atrioventricular interval optimization after biventricular pacing: echo/Doppler vs. impedance plethysmography [abstract]. Pacing Clin Electrophysiol 2000; 23(4):590.

43. Vrushad RB, Fayn E, Clark W, et al. Non-invasive monitoring of hemodynamic changes during dobutamine stress echocardiographic testing using impedance cardiography (ICG). In: Ellestad MH, Amsterdam EA, editors. Exercise testing new concepts of the new century. Boston: Kluwer Academic Publishers; 2002. p. 127–36.

44. Silver MA, Lazzara D, Slaughter M, et al. Thoracic bioimpedance accurately determines cardiac output in patients with left ventricular assist devices [abstract]. J Card Fail 1999;5(Suppl 1):38.

45. Defaye P, Petit L, Vanzetto G, et al. Optimization of dual chamber pacers programming by thoracic electrical bio-impedance (about 34 cases). Pacing Clin Electrophysiol 1993;16:193 [abstract].

46. Ovsyshcher I, Katz A, Bondy C, et al. Thoracic impedance measurements as a method for assessment of cardiac output in pacemaker patients. Pacing Clin Electrophysiol 1993;16:180 [abstract].

47. Kindermann M, Frohlig G, Doerr T, et al. Optimizing the AV delay in DDD pacemaker patients with high degree AV block: mitral valve Doppler versus impedance cardiography. Pacing Clin Electrophysiol 1997;20:2453–62.

48. Schwaab B, Frohlig G, Alexander C, et al. Influence of right ventricular stimulation site on left ventricular function in atrial synchronous ventricular pacing. J Am Coll Cardiol 1999;33:317–23.

49. Belott P. Bioimpedance in the pacemaker clinic. AACN Clin Issues 1999;10:414–8.

50. Crystal E, Ovsyshcher IE. Cardiac output-based versus empirically programmed AV interval—how different are they? Europace 1999;1:121–5.

51. Hayes DL, Hayes SN, Hyberger LK, et al. Atrioventricular interval optimization after biventricular pacing: echo/Doppler vs. impedance plethysmography. Europace 2000;1(Suppl D):108 [abstract].

52. Adachi H, Hiratsuji T, Sakurai S, et al. Impedance cardiography and quantitative tissue Doppler echocardiography for evaluating the effect of cardiac resynchronization therapy: a case report. J Cardiol 2003;42:37–42.

53. Tse H, Yu C, Park E, et al. Impedance cardiography for atrioventricular interval optimization during permanent left ventricular pacing. Pacing Clin Electrophysiol 2003;26:189–91.

54. Braun MU, Schnabel A, Rauwolf T, et al. Impedance cardiography as a noninvasive technique for atrioventricular interval optimization in cardiac resynchronization therapy. J Interv Card Electrophysiol 2005;13:223–9.

55. Gimbel JR. Method and demonstration of direct confirmation of response to cardiac resynchronization therapy via preimplant temporary biventricular pacing and impedance cardiography. Am J Cardiol 2005;96:874–6.

56. Heinroth KM, Elster M, Nuding S, et al. Impedance cardiography: a useful and reliable tool in optimization of cardiac resynchronization devices. Europace 2007;9(9):744–50.

57. Nollert G, Reichart B. Registration of thoracic electrical bioimpedance for early diagnosis of rejection after heart transplantation. J Heart Lung Transplant 1993;12:832–6.

58. Suttner S, Schollhorn T, Boldt J, et al. Noninvasive assessment of cardiac output using thoracic electrical bioimpedence in hemodynamically stable and unstable patients after cardiac surgery: a comparison with pulmonary artery thermodilution. Intensive Care Med 2006;32:2053–8.

Usefulness of B-type Natriuretic Peptide Levels in Predicting Hemodynamic and Clinical Decompensation

Pam R. Taub, MD[a],*, Lori B. Daniels, MD, MAS[a],
Alan S. Maisel, MD[a],[b]

KEYWORDS

- BNP • Pulmonary congestion
- Heart failure • Decompensation

There are more than 3 million heart failure (HF)-related admissions annually in the United States, and approximately 35% of these admitted patients subsequently have HF-related deaths or readmissions within 60 days.[1-3] Improving methods of assessing preclinical decompensation should be important in reducing HF-related morbidity and mortality.

Natriuretic peptide (NP) levels (ie, B-type natriuretic peptide [BNP] and N-terminal pro BNP [NT-proBNP]) have become a mainstay in the diagnosis or exclusion of acute HF.[4] Emerging evidence suggests that NP levels also might be valuable adjuncts in both treatment monitoring and assessment for possible clinical decompensation.[5-9] Patients who have chronic HF often are on a tenuous portion of the pressure–volume curve, and small volume shifts can mean the difference between pulmonary edema and renal failure. These subtleties often are difficult to discern with clinical examination and chest radiographs. Because BNP usually correlates with pulmonary capillary wedge pressure (PCWP),[10] it should be useful for detecting early subclinical congestion, and this identification can help preventing acute clinical decompensation.

DECOMPENSATION IS RELATED TO PULMONARY CONGESTION

With the increasing use of implantable defibrillators and beta-blockers, pulmonary congestion, rather than low cardiac output, is becoming the leading cause of hospital admissions and death in patients who have HF. In the Vasodilatation in the Management of Acute Congestive Heart Failure trial, the mean wedge pressure of patients admitted for HF was high (25–30 mm Hg), and they tended to have a preserved cardiac index.[11] Similarly, in the Acute Decompensated Heart Failure National Registry of more than 100,000 patients, only 3% of patients admitted with decompensated HF had evidence of low cardiac output with a systolic blood pressure lower than 90 mm Hg.[12]

Previous studies also have shown that high PCWP at discharge is a poor prognostic indicator. In the Evaluation Study of Congestive Heart Failure and Pulmonary Artery Catheterization Effectiveness trial, PCWP was an important predictor of 6-month postdischarge survival.[13] In an observational study of patients hospitalized for decompensated HF, a reduction of PCWP to below 16 mm Hg at discharge was associated with decreased 2-year mortality, whereas a cardiac index above 2.6 L/min/m^2 was not associated with improved outcome (**Fig. 1**).[14] Thus the wedge pressure is an important diagnostic and therapeutic target.

The cascade that ultimately leads to pulmonary congestion often begins with an increased blood

[a] University of California San Diego Medical Center, San Diego, CA, USA
[b] Veterans Affairs Medical Center, San Diego, CA, USA
* Corresponding author. Division of Cardiology, University of California, San Diego Medical Center, 200 West Arbor Drive, San Diego, CA 92103-8411.
E-mail address: ptaub@ucsd.edu (P.R. Taub).

Heart Failure Clin 5 (2009) 169–175
doi:10.1016/j.hfc.2008.11.009
1551-7136/08/$ – see front matter © 2009 Elsevier Inc. All rights reserved

volume leading to increased left ventricular end-diastolic pressure and elevated PCWP. High pressures reflected into the lungs lead to redistribution in the pulmonary vascular bed with subsequent interstitial edema followed by alveolar edema. This pulmonary congestion is manifested clinically by symptoms of shortness of breath and orthopnea and by lung rales on examination. Eventually, increased pulmonary artery pressure may lead to elevated right ventricular and right atrial pressures. This increased pressure causes clinical symptoms of systemic, or right-sided, congestion such as jugular venous distension and peripheral edema (**Fig. 2**). As shown in **Fig. 3**, in a study of 32 patients who had chronic HF implanted with a hemodynamic monitor, there was a rise in measures of volume overload up to 7 days before hospitalization for acute decompensated HF.[15] Thus there is an important preclinical window in which congestion is masked; if congestion is detected and addressed during this window, hospitalizations may decrease (see **Fig. 3**).

Congestion secondary to an increase in left ventricular wall stress (especially diastolic) also is accompanied by rapid synthesis and release of BNP from the cardiac myocyte.[16] Resolution of clinical congestion occurs before the restoration of normal cardiovascular hemodynamics. One reason patients who clinically seem to be euvolemic on discharge decompensate after discharge may be that their subclinical hemodynamic derangements are still present.[3]

CONGESTION IS DIFFICULT TO ASCERTAIN ON PHYSICAL EXAMINATION

Even in the best of hands, establishing the diagnosis of HF may be clinically challenging. Physical examination findings such as rales, increased jugular venous pressure, and edema are specific but not sensitive for elevated cardiac filling pressures.[17] In one recent study, the third heart sound was 92% specific for HF but was only 41% sensitive.[18] Also, in a subset of patients who have HF, there is a discrepancy between jugular venous pressure and PCWP. Some patients may have a predominantly right-sided HF with pulmonary hypertension and may have elevated jugular venous pressure but a normal lung examination. Conversely, patients who have systolic HF but intact right heart function may have high wedge pressure and low central venous pressure. In addition, radiographic findings often lag behind clinical findings and thus are not always useful in diagnosing acute decompensation or clinical improvement.[19] Thus, hemodynamic abnormalities such as elevated PCWP do not always correlate with clinical symptoms and signs and may go unrecognized until patients present with decompensation. The lack of sensitivity of the clinical findings in establishing the diagnosis of pulmonary congestion also may make it difficult to ascertain the point in the clinical course of treatment when euvolemia has been established.

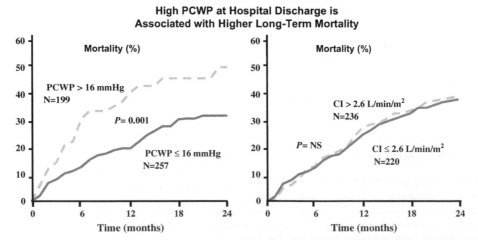

Fig. 1. In an observational study of patients hospitalized for decompensated HF, reduction of PCWP to less than 16 mm Hg was associated with reduced mortality, whereas the cardiac index was not associated with mortality in this patient group. CI, cardiac index. (*Data from* Fonarow GC, Stevenson LW, Steimle AE, et al. Persistently high left ventricular filling pressures predict mortality despite angiotensin converting enzyme inhibition in advanced heart failure. Circulation 1994;90:1–488; with permission. *Courtesy of* M. Gheorgiade, MD, Chicago, IL.)

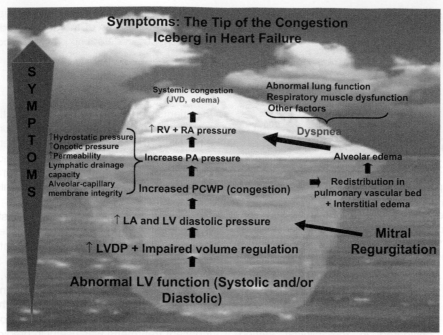

Fig. 2. The tip of the iceberg represents the late clinical symptoms of congestion that occur after a subclinical period of days to weeks during which the PCWP has been elevated and difficult to detect by clinical examination alone. LA, left atrial, LV, left ventricular, LVDP, left ventricular diastolic pressure, JVD, jugular vein distension, RA, right atrial, RV, right ventricular. (*Courtesy of* M. Gheorgiade, MD, Chicago, IL.)

USE OF NATRIURETIC PEPTIDES TO ASSESS CONGESTION

Because NP levels have a short half-life and can change dynamically based on a reduction or increase in left ventricular wall stress, they offer insight into a patient's clinical status at multiple levels. BNP can be particularly useful as an early marker of congestion because BNP levels often correlate with PCWP.[10] In a pilot study of 20 patients admitted for acute HF with clinical features of volume overload, a Swan-Ganz catheter was placed and BNP measurements were taken serially. With treatment, BNP levels correlated with decreased PCWP (**Fig. 4**). In fact, consistent with the half-life of BNP being only 20 minutes, decreases in BNP levels at a rate of 35 to 50 pg/mL/h were achieved in patients showing a clinical response to diuresis. In contrast, patients who did not respond to treatment (many of whom had end-stage HF) did not have a decrease in BNP levels.[10] Importantly, BNP levels do not instantaneously reflect changes in PCWP; thus BNP is best used to follow trends, and one must be careful not to overinterpret any individual time-point.[3]

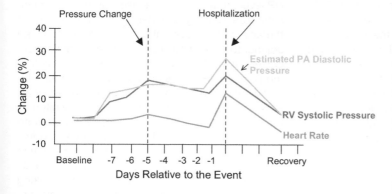

Fig. 3. An implantable hemodynamic monitor was used to assess right ventricular and pulmonary artery diastolic pressures and revealed a gradual rise in these pressures several days before hospitalizations for acute HF. PA, pulmonary artery; RV, right ventricular. (*From* Adamson PB, Magalski A, Braunschweig F, et al. Ongoing right ventricular hemodynamics in heart failure: clinical value of measurements derived from an implantable monitoring system. J Am Coll Cardiol 2003;41:565; with permission. *Courtesy of* M. Gheorgiade, MD, Chicago, IL.)

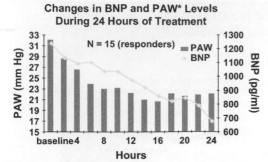

Changes in BNP and PAW* Levels During 24 Hours of Treatment

N = 15 (responders)

*Pulmonary artery wedge.

Fig. 4. BNP levels and pulmonary artery pressures are correlated and decline with treatment. (*From* Kazanegra B, Chang V, Garcia A, et al. A rapid test for B-type natriuretic peptide correlates with falling wedge pressures in patients treated for decompensated heart failure: a pilot study. J Cardiac Fail 2001;7(1):21–9; with permission.)

Multiple factors that can confound NP levels must be considered in the clinical setting. Advanced age, renal dysfunction, pulmonary embolism, atrial fibrillation, and high output states (such as sepsis, cirrhosis, or hyperthyroidism) can cause elevated BNP levels.[20] Obesity, flash pulmonary edema, acute mitral regurgitation, cardiac tamponade, and pericardial constriction can result in BNP levels lower than expected.[20]

There often is intra-individual variability in BNP levels. In a small study of 45 patients who had clinically stable HF, there was intra-individual variability of 14.6% over 1 hour and 28.4% over 1 week. The results of this study suggest that an increase from baseline of at least 50% for NT-proBNP and 66% for BNP is needed to signify a significant change in clinical status.[21]

In addition, BNP does not correlate with PCWP in some clinical settings. In right-sided failure from cor pulmonale, a high BNP level does not reflect elevated PCWP. Scenarios in which BNP levels are low despite elevated PCWP include acute mitral regurgitation, when the increase in PCWP is upstream from the left ventricle, and "flash" pulmonary edema, when there may not have been enough time for BNP to be synthesized.[22] Also, in patients who have noncardiogenic causes of shock such as sepsis, BNP levels do not correlate strongly with PCWP, although they have a strong correlation with ultimate prognosis.[23,24]

Emerging clinical tools to detect early congestion include measuring intrathoracic impedance. In small pilot trials, the use of biventricular implantable cardioverter-defibrillators with built-in technology to measure intrathoracic impedance was associated with decreased hospital admissions

for HF.[25,26] In the future, combined use of BNP along with measures of thoracic impedance may be synergistic in detecting preclinical congestion.

NATRIURETIC PEPTIDE ASSESSMENT IN THE INPATIENT SETTING

In patients who have decompensated HF, the BNP level can be thought of as having two components: a baseline "dry" component when patients are optivolemic and at their dry weight, and a "wet" component, or the additional BNP produced in patients who have volume overload, which reflects increased hemodynamic stress.[20,22]

Cheng and colleagues[8] were the first to report that patients who had a drop in BNP level during their hospitalization had a much better short-term prognosis than patients whose BNP level increased or stayed the same. Similarly, in a study of 223 patients hospitalized for decompensated HF, Logeart and colleagues[27] found that predischarge BNP (which reflects the effect of intensive inpatient treatment) was useful in predicting postdischarge outcomes (**Fig. 5**). A high predischarge BNP (>700 pg/mL), which suggested that the patient had significant subclinical pulmonary congestion, was an independent predictor of readmission and death. Patients who had lower discharge BNP levels (<350 pg/mL), which may reflect an optivolemic state and/or a less advanced stage of HF, had a lower incidence of death and readmission. In a small study of 116 patients, Dokinasish and colleagues[28] found that use of predischarge BNP levels is more cost effective than using Doppler-echocardiographic indices of elevated left ventricular filling pressure in predicting future HF-related adverse events.

NATRIURETIC PEPTIDE LEVELS IN THE OUTPATIENT SETTING

NP levels may prove to be useful in the outpatient setting as a surrogate to help guide titration of drug therapy, and NP levels already may be useful as an adjunct for detecting subclinical decompensation. Observations from several studies indicated that monitoring NP levels in outpatients could ultimately improve outcomes. In the Valsartan Heart Failure trial, treatment with valsartan resulted in decreased BNP levels.[5] Similarly, Tsumatamoto and colleagues[6] showed that treatment with spironolactone reduced BNP levels, and this reduction correlated with improved ejection fraction. Treatment with beta-blockers in patients already taking angiotensin-converting enzyme (ACE) inhibitors also resulted in decreased BNP levels.[7] These reductions in BNP likely stem from neurohormonal

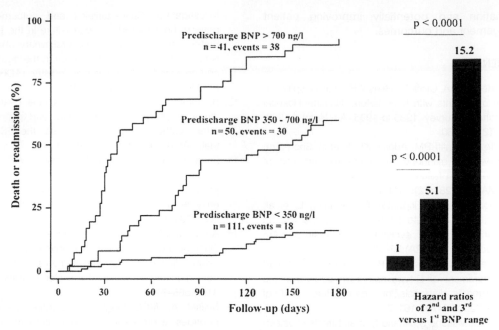

Fig. 5. Predischarge BNP levels higher than 700 pg/mL were associated with higher rates of readmission or death than predischarge BNP levels lower than 350 pg/mL. (*From* Logeart D, Thabut G, Jourdain P, et al. Predischarge B-type natriuretic peptide assay for identifying patients at high risk of re-admission after decompensated heart failure. J Am Coll Cardiol 2004;43(4):639; with permission.)

blockade and from the positive effects of these drugs on ventricular remodeling. These observations have led to studies in which BNP levels were used to titrate drug therapy in patients who had chronic HF.

In the Systolic Heart Failure Treatment Supported by BNP (STARS BNP) trial, all 220 patients were treated with optimal medical therapy consisting of beta-blockers, ACE inhibitors, and diuretics but were assigned randomly to have their treatment guided by standard guidelines (the clinical group) or by a goal of decreasing BNP to less than 100 pg/mL (the BNP group).[29] The authors found that patients in the BNP-guided group received higher mean doses of beta-blockers and ACE inhibitors, and the BNP-guided strategy resulted in reduced risk of HF-related adverse outcomes.[29] A BNP-guided strategy did not improve outcomes significantly, however, in the Strategies for Tailoring Advanced Heart Failure Regimens in the Outpatient Setting: Brain Natriuretic Peptide Versus the Clinical Congestion Score (STARBRIGHT) trial of 160 outpatients, which targeted a BNP level of two times less than the predischarge BNP.[30] The difference between the results of these two trials may stem from STARBRIGHT using a higher BNP target and enrolling sicker patients.[20] Both the STARS BNP and the STARBRIGHT trials were small, and the results of trials such as the Placebo-controlled

Randomized Study of the Selective A1 Adenosine Receptor Antagonist KW-3902 for Patients Hospitalized with Acute HF and Volume Overload to Assess Treatment Effect on Congestion and Renal Function and the BNP-Assisted Treatment to Lessen Serial Cardiac Readmission and Death are awaited.

Traditional methods of monitoring congestion such as daily weights are confounded by multiple variables such as patient food and fluid intake and the time of day when measurements are taken. Home BNP testing may emerge as a modality to monitor a patient's level of congestion and to help titrate the medication regimen in the outpatient setting.

SUMMARY

Pulmonary congestion is difficult to diagnose, whether in an individual who has new-onset dyspnea, a patient who has known HF and a possible exacerbation, or an outpatient whose HF treatment may not have been adequate. Assessing when euvolemia has been achieved following treatment of congestion also is challenging. Tools such as the NPs are important adjuncts to the physical examination and radiography and often may obviate the need for invasive hemodynamic assessment while providing important prognostic information and potentially improving patient management and outcomes.

REFERENCES

1. Haldeman GA, Croft JB, Giles WH, et al. Hospitalization of patients with heart failure: National Hospital Discharge Survey, 1985 to 1995. Am Heart J 1999; 137(2):352–60.
2. Cuffe MS, Califf RM, Adams KF Jr, et al. Short-term intravenous milrinone for acute exacerbation of chronic heart failure: a randomized controlled trial. JAMA 2002;287(12):1541–7.
3. Gheorghiade M, Filippatos G, De Luca L, et al. Congestion in acute heart failure syndromes: an essential target of evaluation and treatment. Am J Med 2006;119(12A):S3–10.
4. Maisel AS, Krishnaswamy P, Nowak RM, et al. Rapid measurement of B-type natriuretic peptide in the emergency diagnosis of heart failure. N Engl J Med 2002;34793:161–7.
5. Latini R, Masson S, Anand I, et al. Effects of valsartan on circulating brain natriuretic peptide and norepinephrine in symptomatic chronic heart failure: the Valsartan Heart Failure Trial (Val-HeFT). Circulation 2002;106(19):2454–8.
6. Tsutamoto T, Wada A, Maeda K, et al. Effect of spironolactone on plasma brain natriuretic peptide in patients with congestive heart failure. J Am Coll Cardiol 2001;37(5):1228–33.
7. Fung JW, Yu CM, Yip G, et al. Effect of beta-blockade (carvedilol or metoprolol) on activation of the renin-angiotensin-aldosterone system and natriuretic peptides in chronic heart failure. Am J Cardiol 2003;92(4):406–10.
8. Cheng V, Kazanagra R, Garcia A, et al. A rapid bedside test for B-type peptide predicts treatment outcomes in patients admitted for decompensated hear failure: a pilot study. J Am Coll Cardiol 2001; 37(2):386–91.
9. Bettencourt P, Ferreira S, Azevedo A, et al. Preliminary data on the potential usefulness of B-type natriuretic peptide levels in predicting outcome after hospital discharge in patients with heart failure. Am J Med 2002;113(3):215–9.
10. Kazanegra R, Cheng V, Garcia A, et al. A rapid test for B-type natriuretic peptide correlates with falling wedge pressure in patients treated for decompensated heart failure: a pilot study. J Card Fail 2001; 7(1):21–9.
11. Publication Committee for the VMAC Investigators. Intravenous nesiritide vs nitroglycerin for treatment of decompensated congestive heart failure: a randomized controlled trial. J Am Med Assoc 2002;287(12):1531–40.
12. Adams KF Jr, Fonarow GC, Emerman CL, et al. For the ADHERE Scientific Advisory Committee and Investigators. Characteristics and outcomes of patients hospitalized for heart failure in the United States: rationale, design and preliminary observations from the first 100,000 cases in the acute decompensated failure national registry (ADHERE). Am Heart J 2005;149(2):209–16.
13. Binanay C, Califf RM, Hasselblad V, et al. Evaluation study of congestive heart failure and pulmonary artery catheterization effectiveness: the ESCAPE trial. JAMA 2005;294(13):1625–33.
14. Fonarow GC, Stevenson LW, Steimle AE, et al. Persistently high left ventricular filling pressures predict mortality despite angiotensin converting enzyme inhibition in advanced heart failure. Circulation 1994;90:1–488.
15. Admason PB, Magalski A, Branunschweig F, et al. Ongoing right ventricular hemodynamics in heart failure: clinical value of measurements from implantable monitoring system. J Am Coll Cardiol 2003; 41(4):565–71.
16. Maisel A, MCCullough PA. Cardiac natriuretic peptides: a proteomic window to cardiac function and clinical management. Rev Cardiovasc Med 2003;4:S3–12.
17. Dao Q, Krishnaswamy P, Kazanegra R, et al. Utility of B-type natriuretic peptide in the diagnosis of congestive heart failure in an urgent-care setting. J Am Coll Cardiol 2001;37(2):379–85.
18. Marcus GM, Gerber IL, McKeown BH, et al. Association between phonocardiographic third and fourth heart sounds and objective measures of left ventricular function. JAMA 2005;293(18):2238–44.
19. Stevenson LW, Perloff JK. The limited reliability of physical signs for estimating hemodynamics in chronic heart failure. JAMA 1989;261(6):884–8.
20. Daniels LB, Maisel AS. Natriuretic peptides. J Am Coll Cardiol 2007;50(25):2357–68.
21. O'Hanlon R, O' Shea P, Ledwidge M, et al. The biologic variability of B-type natriuretic peptide and N-terminal pro-B-type natriuretic peptide in stable heart failure patients. J Card Fail 2007;13(1):50–5.
22. Maisel A. Use of BNP levels in monitoring hospitalized heart failure patients with heart failure. Heart Fail Rev 2003;8(4):339–44.
23. Forfia PR, Watkins SP, Rame JE, et al. Relationship between B-type natriuretic peptides and pulmonary capillary wedge pressure in the intensive care unit. J Am Coll Cardiol 2005;45(10):1667–71.
24. Tung RH, Garcia C, Morss Am, et al. Utility of B-type natriuretic peptide for the evaluation of intensive care unit shock. Crit Care Med 2004;32(8):1643–7.
25. Maines M, Catanzariti D, Cemin C, et al. Usefulness of intrathoracic fluids accumulation monitoring with an implantable biventricular defibrillator in reducing hospitalizations in patients with heart failure: a case-control study. J Interv Card Electrophysiol 2007; 19(3):201–7.

26. Ypenburg C, Bax JJ, van der Wall EE, et al. Intra-thoracic impedance monitoring to predict decompensated heart failure. Am J Cardiol 2007;99(4): 554–7.

27. Logeart D, Thabut G, Jourdain P, et al. Predischarge B-type natriuretic peptide assay for identifying patients at high risk of re-admission after decompensated heart failure. J Am Coll Cardiol 2004; 43(4):635–41.

28. Dokainish H, Zoghbi WA, Lakkis, et al. Incremental predictive power of B-type natriuretic peptide and tissue Doppler echocardiography in the prognosis of patients with congestive heart failure. J Am Coll Cardiol 2005;45(8):1223–6.

29. Jourdain P, Jondeau G, Funck F, et al. Plasma brain natriuretic peptide-guided therapy to improve outcome in heart failure. The STARS-BNP Multicenter Study. J Am Coll Cardiol 2007; 49(16):1733–9.

30. Shan MR, Califf RM, Nohira A, et al. STARBRITE: a randomized pilot trial of BNP-guided therapy in patients with advanced heart failure. Presented at: American Heart Association Scientific Sessions. Chicago, November 12–15, 2006.

Assessment of Left Ventricular Systolic Function by Echocardiography

Martin G. St. John Sutton, MBBS, FRCP*, Ted Plappert, CVT,
Hind Rahmouni, MD

KEYWORDS

- Echocardiography • Remodeling • Heart failure
- Systolic function

Echocardiography serves an extremely important role in the diagnosis and management of patients with heart failure (HF). The various stages of structural and functional changes that constitute progressive left ventricle (LV) remodeling have all been characterized by two-dimensional echocardiography. In addition, echocardiography has defined the transition from compensated hypertrophy to LV dilatation and progression to end-stage HF. Echocardiography has also played an important role in clinical HF trials of β-adrenergic blocking agents and angiotensin-converting enzyme inhibitors and angiotensin receptor blockers and demonstrated their efficacy in HF. Echocardiography has been regarded as the single most useful diagnostic tool in the overall management of patients with HF.

EPIDEMIOLOGY OF HEART FAILURE

There is an estimated 25 to 30 million subjects with HF worldwide, and with an additional half a million new cases diagnosed each year in the United States alone. HF increases with age, and by the year 2035 there will be more than 75 million subjects over 75 years old in the United States so that as longevity increases, HF will increase to epidemic proportions. Already HF constitutes the most prevalent ICD coding for hospital discharge diagnosis in patients older than 65 years. The current prevalence of HF, its impact on employment status, combined with the poor quality of life, the adverse long-term prognosis, and the prohibitive health costs have resulted in HF becoming a high-priority health care initiative worldwide.

SYSTOLIC VERSUS DIASTOLIC HEART FAILURE

Approximately 35% to 50% of patients presenting with typical symptoms of dyspnea caused by pulmonary congestion and clinical signs of HF for the first time have preserved LV ejection fraction, and this has been variously called diastolic HF or HF with preserved LV function (ejection fraction >50%).[1,2] Clinical examination of the cardiovascular system does not reliably distinguish between systolic and diastolic HF (ejection fraction <50%), although chronic systemic hypertension and female gender are more commonly associated with diastolic than with systolic HF.[3] There are several reasons why diastolic HF took so long to be recognized as a discrete entity, not least of which was the notion that diastolic HF was regarded as relatively benign, difficult to define, and for which there was no specific therapy. Diastolic HF has subsequently been shown to have a significant morbidity and mortality, albeit lower than that associated with systolic HF.[4] The etiology in more than two thirds of systolic HF patients (left ventricular ejection fraction [LVEF] <50%) is chronic ischemic heart disease caused by epicardial coronary stenoses or occlusions.

University of Pennsylvania Medical Center, Philadelphia, PA, USA
* Corresponding author. Division of Cardiology, Department of Medicine, University of Pennsylvania Medical Center, 3400 Spruce Street, Philadelphia, PA 19104.
E-mail address: suttonm@mail.med.upenn.edu (M. G. St. John Sutton).

Heart Failure Clin 5 (2009) 177–190
doi:10.1016/j.hfc.2008.11.010
1551-7136/08/$ – see front matter

heartfailure.theclinics.com

The etiology in the remaining patients with systolic HF includes primary-idiopathic cardiomyopathy, hypertension, valvular heart disease, and myocarditis.

This article describes the various echocardiographic techniques that are both universally available and currently used routinely in the diagnosis and management of systolic HF. Echocardiography can be used to triage patients with systolic HF to optimize individual therapy to devices, surgery, or pharmacologic interventions. Brief mention is made of some clinical trials in HF that have used echocardiographic parameters as end points and of some novel technologies that include three-dimensional echocardiographic imaging and endocardial tracking algorithms that provide insight into global and regional myocardial strain, strain rate, and function.

LEFT VENTRICLE INTERNAL DIMENSIONS

M-mode echocardiography was the original noninvasive method for assessing LV size, LV mass, and contractile function (**Fig. 1**). Combined either with continuous LV pressure or cuff-systolic blood pressure measurements, M-mode echocardiographic estimates of LV dimensions and wall thicknesses enabled exploration of wall stress and strain as determinants of LV architecture and contractile function, myocardial relaxation, and mural and cavity mechanics in HF.[5,6] Moreover, M-mode echo measurements of LV dimensions and wall thicknesses have been used extensively to assess LV mass in large, randomized-controlled clinical trials of hypertensive populations.[7–9] These

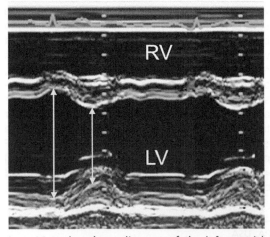

Fig. 1. M-mode echocardiogram of the left ventricle (LV) showing the septum and posterior wall. The arrows represent measurements of internal dimensions at end-diastole (*left arrow*) and at end-systole (*right arrow*).

studies have provided normative data; demonstrated the close relationship between LV size, mass, and body height; and aided in elucidating the different patterns of LV hypertrophy during eccentric versus concentric remodeling (**Fig. 2**).[8,9] M-mode echo continues to be used extensively in randomized clinical trials to quantify regression of LV hypertrophy following interventions to assess the efficacy of a variety of new pharmacologic antihypertensive agents and treatment regimens.

The major advantage of M-mode echocardiography is the high temporal resolution caused by the sampling frequency of 1000 cycles per second. The disadvantages of M-mode are that it assumes that the LV contracts concentrically and there are no regional LV wall motion abnormalities, that the LV wall thickness is uniform, and that contraction of the LV minor axis dimension sampled with two-dimensional echo guidance is truly representative of the whole ventricle. Furthermore, estimation of LV volumes from M-mode assumes fixed LV geometry and a fixed cavity short-to-long axis ratio that results in spuriously high ejection fractions. In systolic HF, the LV is almost invariably enlarged and this is associated with change in shape, and deviation from the normal axis ratio may confound quantification of LV volume and mass even in serial echoes over time.

LEFT VENTRICULAR VOLUMES

A number of different algorithms and geometric models have been used to assess LV end-diastolic and end-systolic volumes from a variety of imaging modalities including two-dimensional echocardiographic images. These echo volumes have been validated against volumes of casts of the LV, postmortem hearts, or MRI.

The LV is bullet-shaped and the recommendations of the American Society of Echocardiology for quantification of LV chamber volumes is Simpson's method of discs,[10] which requires manual digitization of the endocardial boundaries ideally from paired biplane images of the near-orthogonal apical four-chamber and the apical two- chamber views (**Fig. 3**). Accurate and reproducible estimates of LV volumes can be obtained, however, from single plane images of either the apical four-chamber or two-chamber views. Both of these correlate closely with biplane volumes, but are numerically different and cannot be used interchangeably with biplane volumes during serial follow-up.[11] Reproducibility of LV volumes varies because it depends on the quality of the echocardiographic images, identification of the

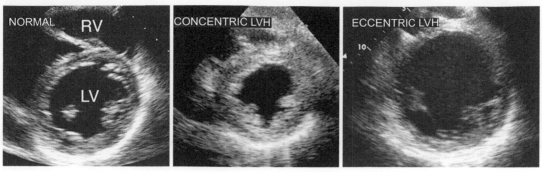

Fig. 2. Dimensional echocardiogram of the LV short axis of a normal heart (*left panel*), of an LV with concentric remodeling *(center panel)*, and an LV with eccentric remodeling *(right panel)*.

endocardial boundaries, and the accuracy of manual digitization of the images (**Fig. 4**). All three of these factors vary from laboratory to laboratory from approximately 5% in busy experienced echo core laboratories to 10% and above in small laboratories where quantitative echocardiography is the exception rather than the rule.

Echocardiographic LV volumes are frequently used in HF trials as "clinical end points" that usually require the services of an experienced quantitative core laboratory because the expected change in LV volume from an intervention may be so small that it may be lost in the signal-to-noise ratio in a routine busy clinical laboratory.[12]

Recently, speckle-tracking technologies have been developed (AutoEF) using artificial intelligence and pattern recognition to facilitate endocardial recognition and provide continuous LV volumes almost instantaneously (**Fig. 5**).[13] Although the AutoEF system software in its current form functions well in normal hearts, it fares less well in the presence of mechanical valve

prostheses or in large hearts with abnormal shape that typify HF.[14] The reproducibility of the automated LV volume estimates was superior to manual digitization as compared with the reproducibility typically obtained in a busy echo core laboratory using two-dimensional quantitative imaging.[14] In the authors' experience, however, automated volume computation systematically underestimated LV volumes calculated both by MRI and by manual digitization because of consistent failure to recognize the endocardium of the lateral wall.[14] Recently engineered software upgrades may improve the accuracy of automated volume quantification in hearts of varying sizes and shapes.

Commercially available software for three-dimensional echo full-volume quantitative analysis of LV volumes has demonstrated closer agreement and less variability than with assessment by two-dimensional when compared with volumes estimated by MRI, which is regarded as the gold standard for LV volume computation.[15]

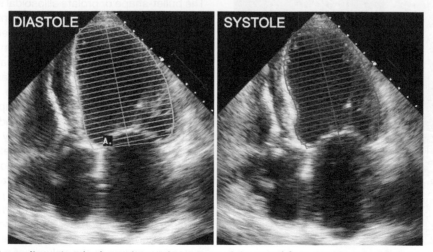

Fig. 3. Paired two-dimensional echocardiographic images of the apical four-chamber view (*left panel*) and apical two-chamber view (*right panel*) showing digitized endocardial boundaries for LV volume computations using Simpson's method.

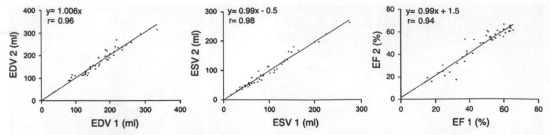

Fig. 4. Interobserver reproducibility of manually digitized LV end-diastolic volumes (EDV), end-systolic volumes (ESV), and ejection fraction (EF).

Independent of the three-dimensional method used for quantification of LV volumes, there are no assumptions regarding LV shape or plane positioning errors with three-dimensional echo, and volumes exhibit less scatter and less interobserver variability (**Fig. 6**). A number of studies have clearly demonstrated that three-dimensional echocardiography is superior to two-dimensional echocardiography for accurate and reproducible estimation of LV volumes.[15] Although three-dimensional echocardiography is being used with increasing frequency nationwide and is acknowledged to be superior to two-dimensional echo for volume quantification, quantitative three-dimensional echocardiography has not yet been used in any randomized interventional clinical HF trials.

The importance of LV volumes resides in the fact that they provide powerful prognostic information pertaining to clinical outcome including mortality, recurrent HF requiring hospital admission, and recurrent myocardial function in patients with LV systolic dysfunction and HF. In a number of post–myocardial infarction and HF trials of patients with LV dysfunction and clinical HF (LVEF <40%), LV end-systolic volume has emerged as the single most important predictor of mortality and new-onset HF necessitating hospital admission.[16] Furthermore, the risk of a serious adverse cardiovascular event, including death, HF, or recurrent myocardial infarction, increases in direct proportion to increase in LV systolic volume (**Fig. 7**).[17] In addition, there is a striking direct relationship between LV volumes and incidence of ventricular arrhythmias[18] in survivors of myocardial infarction with residual LV dysfunction. The strong correlations between LV end-systolic volume and ventricular ectopy and between LV end-systolic volume and potentially life-threatening ventricular tachycardia persisted for at least 2 years postinfarction (**Fig. 8**).[18]

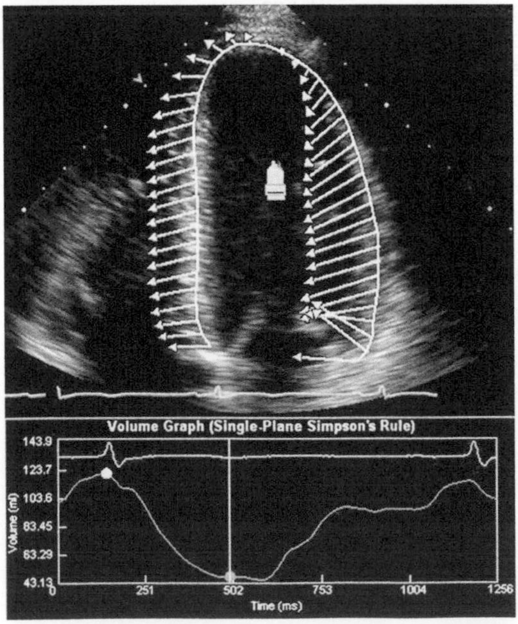

LEFT VENTRICLE SHAPE

The bullet-shape or prolate ellipsoidal shape of the normal human LV is conserved from infancy to old age. In systolic HF, however, the LV enlarges and as it does so the cavity shape becomes progressively distorted by the disproportionately greater increase in short axis than in long axis (**Fig. 9**), and this LV distortion is predictive of adverse clinical outcome.[19] Change in LV shape has been estimated echocardiographically and is usually expressed as an index of sphericity defined as the ratio of the LV short-axis diameter/LV long-axis length. Cavity shape becomes more spherical as the LV enlarges, because a sphere accommodates the greatest volume per unit perimeter of any geometric configuration. An alternative echocardiographic method for estimating LV cavity shape at end-diastole and end-systole is by indexing cavity volume to the volume of a sphere with a diameter equal to LV cavity length measured in the apical four-chamber view.[20] As LV volume

Fig. 5. Velocity vector imaging uses speckle tracking to provide automated endocardial definition and LV volume computation.

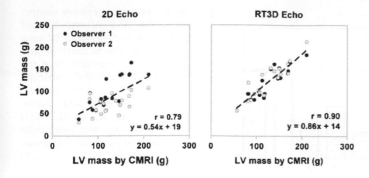

Fig. 6. Agreement between LV mass calculated from two-dimensional echocardiography and cardiac MRI (CMRI) that has become the gold standard (*left panel*), and agreement between LV mass by real-time three-dimensional echocardiography (RT3D) (*right panel*) and CMRI. Three-dimensional RT echo has a greater correlation coefficient with CMRI than two-dimensional echo and with less variability. (*From* Mor-Avi V, Sugeng L, Weinert L, et al. Fast measurement of left ventricular mass with real-time three-dimensional echocardiography: comparison with magnetic resonance imaging. Circulation 2004;110:1814–8; with permission.)

increases, the shape-sphericity index increases toward unity, which would represent a perfect sphere. Change in cavity shape to a more spherical configuration is associated with poor outcome that persists even after adjusting for LV volumes.

LEFT VENTRICLE GLOBAL FUNCTION
Ejection Fraction

The most frequent assessment of LV function is ejection fraction, which can be derived as the difference between end-diastolic and end-systolic volumes, which represents stroke volume, expressed as a percentage of end-diastolic volume:

$$EDV - ESV = SV \text{ (stroke volume)}$$

$$LVEF = SV/EDV \times 100\%$$

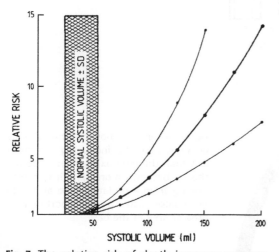

Fig. 7. The relative risk of death increases exponentially with increasing LV end-systolic volume. This relationship demonstrates the importance of end-systolic volume for early risk stratification. (*From* White HD, Norris RM, Brown MA, et al. Left ventricular end-systolic volume as the major determinant of survival after recovery from myocardial infarction. Circulation 1987;76:44–51; with permission.)

LVEF describes global left ventricular cavity function, and normal values independent of age or gender are greater than 55%. Although LVEF is dimensionless and exquisitely sensitive to perturbations in loading conditions, it has been shown to be a powerful predictor of clinical outcome in patients with and without HF from valvular heart disease and ischemic and idiopathic LV dysfunction. LVEF has been used to define inclusion and exclusion criteria for multiple randomized clinical trials assessing the efficacy of angiotensin-converting enzyme inhibitors, angiotensin receptor blockers, vasodilators and β-adrenergic receptor blockers, and resynchronization devices in patients with HF.[21–24] LVEF is used to stratify risk and appropriateness of HF patients for adjuvant device therapies that include epicardial constraint, biventricular pacing, mitral valve replacement, ventricular-assist devices, cardiac transplantation, internal cardiac defibrillators, and novel pharmacologic interventions.[21–25]

Although LVEF should be calculated from end-diastolic and end-systolic volumes obtained from digitized paired biplane orthogonal apical images, visual estimates of LVEF by experienced level three trained echocardiologists correlate very closely with those obtained from digitized images and are used extensively in clinical practice for risk stratification, clinical decision making, and interventional therapies.

Left Ventricle Fractional Shortening

Linear measurements of the LV short-axis dimensions at end-diastole and end-systole by two-dimensional directed M-mode echo can be used to estimate fractional systolic LV shortening as an index of contractile function as:

$$\%\Delta LVD = (LVED - LVES/LVED) \times 100\%$$

The percent change in M-mode measurements of LV minor axis dimensions, although providing

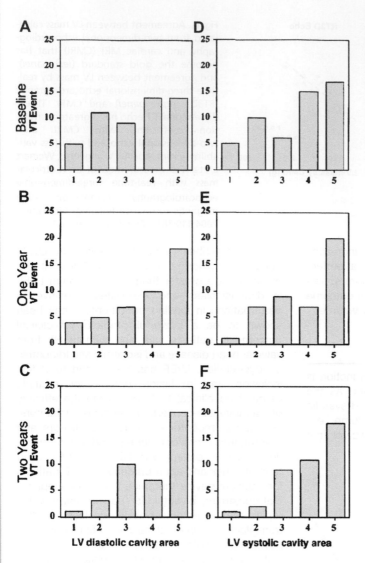

Fig. 8. The relationships between ventricular tachycardia and LV end-diastolic (A-C) cavity area and size and LV end-systolic (D-F) cavity size at baseline, at 1 year, and at 2 years indicating that the incidence of life-threatening ventricular tachycardia increases in direct proportion to LV size. (From St. John Sutton M, Lee D, Rouleau JL, et al. Left ventricular remodeling and ventricular arrhythmias after myocardial infarction. Circulation 2003;107:2577–82; with permission.)

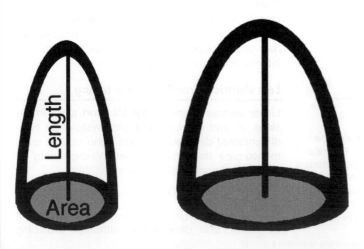

Fig. 9. Schematic showing that the LV enlarges more by increasing the short axis than the long axis and in so doing, the LV becomes more spherical, transitioning from a prolate ellipse at left to an ellipse with a disproportionately greater area at the base.

some information about LV function, is often confounded when regional variation in function or abnormal septal motion are present. Although the same caution is required when interpreting mid-wall fractional shortening, which requires measurement of LV wall thickness, mid-wall fractional shortening is useful in detecting LV systolic dysfunction in patients with LV hypertrophy.[26]

Regional Left Ventricle Function

Detection of regional variation in myocardial function at rest can be demonstrated as decreased regional myocardial thickening, and reduced endocardial-wall motion during systole provides insight into the etiology of HF. Regional variation in LV function not apparent at rest can be unveiled by stress testing with treadmill exercise, dobutamine, or Persantine in HF patients in conjunction with echocardiographic imaging using currently available conventional protocols. The LV is divided into 17 myocardial segments, similar to the prior 16-segment model except for the apical cap (segment 17), which represents the most distal apical myocardium that extends beyond the LV cavity (**Fig. 10**). The rationale of the stress test in patients with HF is to establish an ischemic etiology, which relies on the fact that coronary flow may be of normal magnitude and distribution at rest with proximal coronary stenosis of 85% to 90%. During exercise stress, a proximal 50% stenosis at the same location may be flow limiting and result in diminished regional myocardial perfusion and blunted contraction. Echocardiographic

imaging is obtained at rest and at peak tolerated stress during which time each of the 17 myocardial segments is analyzed for the extent of systolic thickening and endocardial motion. Normal regional wall thickening is graded 1, hypokinesis is graded 2, akinesis is graded 3, and dyskinesis is graded 4. A wall motion score index is determined as the sum of all scores divided by the number of analyzable segments.[10] This echocardiographic wall motion score index provides information about the location, size, and transmurality of the infarction and how extensive is the region of border zone myocardium at risk.[10]

Left Ventricle Mass

Calculation of left ventricular mass is most frequently obtained using M-mode echocardiography for which measurement of LV cavity diameter, LV posterior wall, and septal thicknesses are required at end-diastole. The algorithm used to calculate LV mass is modeled on prolate ellipsoidal geometry and uniform wall thickness in both short and long axes. This allows calculation of the volume of two ellipses, one with the total volume based on the epicardial surface and the second ellipse (cavity volume) based on the endocardial surface of the LV. Subtraction of end-diastolic cavity volume from the total volume of the epicardial ellipse and multiplying this by the density of muscle (1.04) provides an approximation of LV muscle mass. Limitations of LV mass estimations include errors in measurements of wall thickness that are amplified by a cube

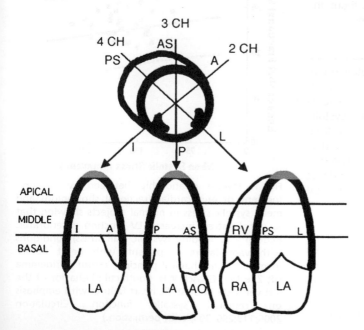

Fig. 10. Schema of the 17-segment model of the LV with the apical cap representing the seventeenth segment. This is the schematic used for assessing regional LV function in which each segment is graded 1 through 4, and a total score is derived by summation of all available scores and by dividing the total by the number of scores evaluated.

function in calculating LV mass. Determinations of LV mass may be confounded in severely dilated hearts with altered cavity geometry and regional wall variation in wall thickness or wall motion.

Relative Wall Thickness and Mass/Volume Ratio

Relative wall thickness (RWT) is defined as:

$$RWT = 2 \times PWTd/LVDd$$

RWT is virtually unchanged throughout life in structurally normal hearts exposed to the normal range of systolic blood pressure (>0.42). Development of systolic HF from systemic hypertension is characterized by concentric remodeling and an increase in RWT, whereas systolic HF caused by chronic severe volume overload from aortic or mitral regurgitation (MR) is associated with eccentric hypertrophic remodeling and reduction in RWT.

In spite of the technical limitations inherent in LV mass calculations from M-mode, two-dimensional and three-dimensional echo, knowledge of LV mass especially as it relates to mass/volume ratio is important, because this ratio remains constant throughout life unless eccentric or concentric remodeling are induced similar to RWT. When the stimulus for remodeling is counterbalanced by therapeutic intervention, the mass/volume ratio reverts toward normal. LV mass in HF patients varies widely from patients who develop severe LV hypertrophy as in nonischemic idiopathic cardiomyopathy to those with ischemic dilated cardiomyopathy who exhibit a limited or inadequate hypertrophic response because of myocytes loss or malfunction and are without the capacity to elaborate contractile proteins.

Wall Stress and Stress-Shortening

Systolic HF is characterized by LV dilatation that initially increases systolic wall stress at the LV endocardium and at the LV mid-wall proportional to the increase in LV size. Meridional end-systolic wall stress (MWS-σ) can be calculated from M-mode echo measurements of LV cavity radius (r), LV wall thickness (h), and cavity length (circumferential stress) with simultaneous direct or indirect (cuff systolic blood pressure) measurement of LV systolic pressure (P).

$$MWS(\sigma) = P \times r/2h(1+h/2r)$$

Circumferential wall stress (CWS-σ) correlates more closely with cavity emptying but requires two-dimensional echocardiography measurement of cavity length.

$$CWS(\sigma) = P \times b/h(1-h/2b)(1-hb/2a)$$

Where "a" and "b" are the major and minor LV cavity axes.

Wall stress is a major determinant of LV cavity architecture, LV hypertrophy, and contractile function. In compensated congestive HF, initial LV dilatation increases wall stress that is transduced by stretch-activated mechanoreceptors that trigger a hypertrophic response by the angiotensin-1 receptor. Hypertrophy results in an increase in LV wall thickness that normalizes wall stress and preserves and stabilizes LV contractile function. There is a strong inverse relationship between systolic wall stress and ejection phase indices including ejection fraction, fractional shortening of the LV internal dimensions, and velocity of circumferential fiber shortening (**Fig. 11**). As systolic wall stress increases, so ejection fraction decreases. This is important from a therapeutic perspective because reducing wall stress is accompanied by improvement in ejection fraction. This is the fundamental principle underlying the use of vasodilator therapy in patients with HF before the onset of irreversible myocardial damage occurs at which point they fall off the normal stress-shortening relationship, leftward and downward. The effects of therapeutic

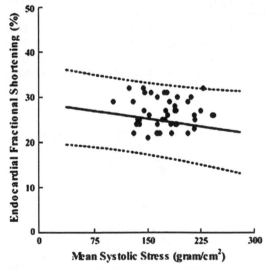

Fig. 11. Inverse relationship between LV function (percent of endocardial fractional shortening) and mean systolic stress in normal subjects showing that as systolic stress increases, LV function deteriorates. Reducing LV loading (systolic wall stress) conditions with vasodilators in patients with heart failure invokes this mechanical principle. (*From* Aurigemma GP, Zile MR, Gaasch WH. Contractile behavior of the left ventricle in diastolic heart failure: with emphasis on regional systolic function. Circulation 2006;113:296–304; with permission.)

interventions aimed at altering LV loading conditions and contractile function can be readily assessed echocardiographically.

The natural history of systolic HF is a progressive deterioration in pump function with the inability to elaborate sufficient hypertrophy to normalize wall stress and prevent the escalation to HF. Assessment of wall stress can be achieved easily by M-mode or two-dimensional measurements of LV cavity radius (diameter/2), wall thickness, and for circumferential wall stress cavity length. In individual patients the slope of the relationship between changes in end-systolic wall stress and end-systolic diameter over a series of perturbations in LV loading conditions provides an index of contractile function that is independent of load.[6] The limitation of calculating wall stress in HF is that the currently used stress equations make the assumption that the material properties of the myocardium are homogeneous and that there are no regional wall motion abnormalities. These conditions are not met in patients with HF of ischemic etiology, who comprise approximately two thirds of all HF patients.

Although estimation of regional and global wall stress assumes that myocardial material properties are homogeneous throughout the LV and calculations become uninterpretable, myocardial strain or deformation can be measured and used as a surrogate for wall stress. Strain is defined in physical terms as the change in myocardial length over resting length:

Strain, $(\epsilon) = \Delta L/L_0$

$\Delta L = (L_t - L_0)$
L_0 = resting length
L_t = length at a specific time "t"

Measurements of myocardial strain can be obtained from tissue Doppler imaging using echocardiography with high temporal and spatial accuracy[27–29] and ideally should be related to the long axis of the myocardial fibers. Echo measurements of myocardial strain correlate closely with strain measurements derived from sonomicrometry crystals and from MRI using myocardial tagging techniques.[30] Tissue Doppler imaging measures myocardial velocity at two locations, whereas sonomicrometry and MRI measure movement between two points. Acquisition of strain measurements from echocardiography is relatively simple, but highly dependent on image and signal quality and consistency. Furthermore, measurement of strain with tissue Doppler imaging is angle dependent and limited to apical echocardiographic images so that only longitudinal strain can be quantified.

An alternative echocardiographic method for assessing myocardial strain that also correlates with LVEF uses speckle tracking technology. This is based on the interference from back-scattered ultrasound waves from neighboring structures that create a speckled pattern that remains stable throughout the cardiac cycle (**Fig. 12**).[31,32] This technique, unlike tissue Doppler imaging, is not angle dependent and enables assessment of radial and circumferential strain in addition to longitudinal strain (**Fig. 13**).[31,32] Strain rate is the rate of change of strain over unit time:

Strain rate $= d\epsilon/dt$

Multidimensional strain and strain rate analyses are attractive because they are based on fundamental physiologic principles of myocardial mechanics, obtainable noninvasively and as such provide insight into the mechanisms of HF, and also serve as a clinical tool for long-term follow-up.

Left Ventricular Pressure-Volume Relations, Left Ventricular Elastance

Further insight into LV chamber function in systolic HF can be obtained by integrating echocardiographic images with pressure or displacement to construct pressure volume loops or pressure-LV short axis area loops with acoustic quantification. From these constructs, single beat estimates of end-systolic pressure-volume relations, stroke work, LV elastance, preload-adjusted maximal power index, and recruitable work can be quantified using two-dimensional echocardiography.[33] Although such studies do clarify current understanding of LV global function in HF, the need for continuous LV or central aortic pressure makes them user-unfriendly methodologies and impractical for widespread use in randomized clinical HF trials, and the same can be said for calculation of systolic wall stress.

Mitral Regurgitation

MR is almost ubiquitous in patients with severe systolic HF regardless of its etiology and the more severe the HF, the greater the likelihood of hemodynamically significant MR. There are different pathoetiologic mechanisms that are distinguishable echocardiographically, although the mitral valve leaflets may be intrinsically normal. The two major causes of MR in HF are ischemic MR that is associated with regional LV wall motion abnormalities and nonischemic cardiomyopathy. Both ischemic and nonischemic HF exhibit progressive LV remodeling and cavity dilatation.

Ischemic MR is associated with a poor prognosis and usually results from ischemia of the

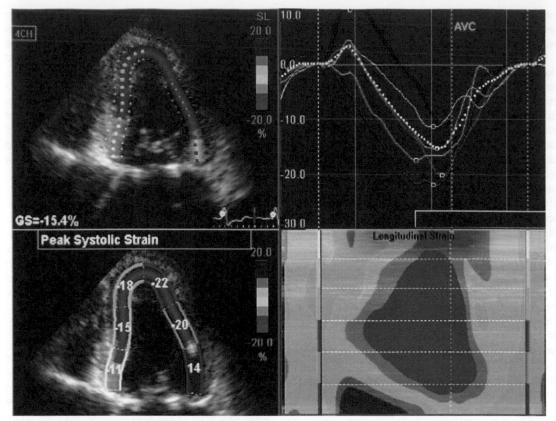

Fig. 12. Peak longitudinal strain obtained using speckle tracking during systolic contraction from six regions of interest that are angle independent and occur almost simultaneously in this normal subject.

papillary muscles or subjacent LV wall, and the severity of MR worsens with the increased demands for exercise stress. Ischemic MR is important to diagnose because it can often be rectified by myocardial revascularization alone, or by revascularization combined with surgical repair of the mitral valve. The diagnosis of ischemic MR can readily be made with transthoracic

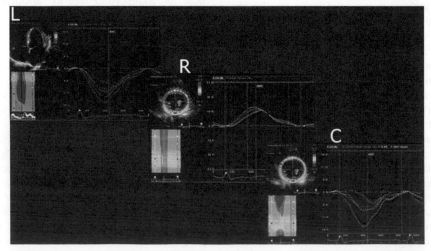

Fig. 13. Schematic showing a plot out of circumferential (C), radial (R), and longitudinal (L) strains from a normal subject in whom there is the usual regional temporal coordination of contraction.

two-dimensional echo Doppler used in conjunction with exercise or pharmacologic stress that exacerbates the degree of MR.

Recognition of MR and assessment of its severity is important because if MR is left untreated it leads to progressive LV dilatation from volume overload that increases wall stress, reduces ejection fraction, and escalates the downward course to HF.[34] MR begets LV dilatation and LV dilatation begets further MR and initiates the remodeling process of progressive deterioration in contractile function that if detected early can be rectified. The severity of MR can often be ameliorated unless irreversible LV dysfunction has supervened. Improvement in MR can be achieved either by reducing LV loading conditions with vasodilators; by surgical repair of the mitral valve; by epicardial restraint devices; or by resynchronization therapy provided that LV dyssynchrony and a prolonged QRS (>120 milliseconds) duration are present.

Color flow Doppler is exquisitely sensitive to MR, allowing detection of even the most trivial MR signal. There are numerous methods for semiquantification of MR by visual estimation of the color flow Doppler jet area and grading severity from 1+ (mild) through 4+ (severe), and true quantification of MR using proximal isovelocity surface area to assess regurgitant volume and effective mitral regurgitant orifice area.

Development of MR in HF of nonischemic etiology is directly related to progressive LV dilatation with disproportionately greater increase in the short axis diameter than in cavity length resulting in a more spherical LV. This change in LV cavity shape separates the two papillary muscles in space with no change in chordal length thereby disrupting normal mitral leaflet area of coaptation causing leaflet tenting and changing the angles that the papillary muscles subtend to the center of the plane of the mitral valve annulus. This distortion of LV that disrupts the normal mitral valve and subvalve apparatus is also accompanied by dilatation of the mitral annulus that facilitates MR. The diagnosis of secondary MR in dilated nonischemic cardiomyopathy is easily established by transthoracic Doppler echocardiography and should be detected early in the course of the remodeling process so that appropriate remedial therapy can be instituted before MR escalates the onset of irreversible LV dysfunction.

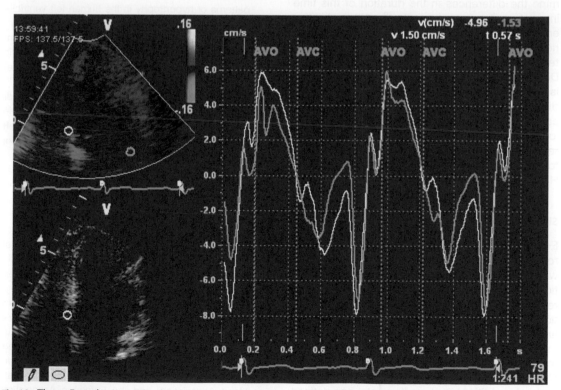

Fig. 14. Tissue Doppler imaging demonstrating continuous myocardial velocities recorded from the basal septum (*yellow*) and basal lateral wall (*green*) from a normal subject. Peak velocities from both regions occur almost simultaneously during LV ejection, indicated by the period between aortic valve opening (AVO) and aortic valve closure (AVC) showing the high degree of temporal coordination of contraction.

Left Ventricle Dyssynchrony

Approximately one third of patients presenting with the symptoms and clinical stigmata of congestive HF have prolonged QRS duration on ECG. QRS duration has been used to establish the presence of LV dyssynchrony. Recent serial echocardiographic studies have demonstrated that cardiac resynchronization therapy (CRT) in patients with advanced HF (New York Heart Association symptom class III/IV) attenuates and more frequently reverses LV remodeling in two thirds of patients.[35–38] The reason postulated for the 30% of nonresponders is a combination of technical problems with the coronary sinus having unfavorable anatomy, or that in spite of the QRS greater than 120 milliseconds there is little evidence for LV dyssynchrony being present. The search for a reliable echocardiographic predictor for LV dyssynchrony and an optimal response to CRT has proved elusive. Initial use of Doppler parameters as predictors of clinical outcome in the PROSPECT randomized trial involved measuring the time interval from the beginning of QRS to both the peak and the onset of peak systolic myocardial velocity (see **Fig. 14**) in the basal two or six myocardial segments to determine the differences in the duration of this time interval between segments.[39] Although this enabled detection of LV dyssynchrony there was no single echo parameter that reliably or consistently predicted response to CRT.[39] The use of Doppler echocardiography and CRT in HF patients is discussed elsewhere in this issue and is not discussed here, other than to mention that echocardiography has characterized the short- and long-term effects of CRT, defined the concept of reversed LV remodeling, and is partly responsible for the role of CRT in patients with symptomatic HF.

SUMMARY

Echocardiography serves an extremely important role in the diagnosis and management of patients with HF. The various stages of structural and functional changes that constitute progressive LV remodeling including changes in loading conditions, hypertrophy, dilatation, cavity shape, mitral annulus, and subvalve apparatus and development of MR are associated with worsening symptoms and quality of life and have all been characterized by two-dimensional echocardiography. In addition, echocardiography has defined the transition from compensated hypertrophy to LV dilatation and progression to end-stage (New York Heart Association class III/IV) HF.

Echocardiography has also played an important role in clinical HF trials of β-adrenergic blocking agents and angiotensin-converting enzyme inhibitor and angiotensin receptor blocker and demonstrated their efficacy in HF. These agents have become standard of care the treatment of HF. It is not surprising that echocardiography has been regarded as the single most useful diagnostic tool in the overall management of patients with HF.

REFERENCES

1. Vasan RS, Levy D. Defining diastolic HF: a call for standardized diagnostic criteria. Circulation 2000; 101:2118–21.
2. Zile MR, Gaasch WH, Carroll JD, et al. Heart failure with a normal ejection fraction: is measurement of diastolic function necessary to make the diagnosis of diastolic HF? Circulation 2001;104:779–82.
3. Kitzman DW, Gardin JM, Gottdiener JS, et al. Importance of HF with preserved systolic function in patients >65 years of age. Am J Cardiol 2001;87:413–9.
4. Smith GL, Masoudi FA, Vaccarino V, et al. Outcomes in HF patients with preserved ejection fraction: mortality, readmission, and functional decline. J Am Coll Cardiol 2003;41:1510–8.
5. Grossman W, Jones D, McLaurin LP. Wall stress and patterns of hypertrophy in the human left ventricle. J Clin Invest 1975;56:14–23.
6. Reichek N, Wilson JR, St. John Sutton M, et al. Noninvasive determination of left ventricular end-systolic stress: validation of the method and initial application. Circulation 1982;65:99–108.
7. Gerdts E, Zabalgoitia M, Bjornstad H, et al. Gender differences in systolic left ventricular function in hypertensive patients with electrocardiographic left ventricular hypertrophy (the LIFE study). Am J Cardiol 2001;87:980–3.
8. Devereux RB, Roman MJ, de Simone G, et al. Relations of left ventricular mass to demographic and hemodynamic variables in American Indians: the Strong Heart Study. Circulation 1997;96:1416–23.
9. Devereux RB, Bella JN, Palmieri V, et al. Left ventricular systolic dysfunction in a biracial sample of hypertensive adults: The Hypertension Genetic Epidemiology Network (Hyper GEN) Study. Hypertension 2001;38:417–23.
10. Lang RM, Bierig M, Devereux RB, et al. A report from the American Society of Echocardiography's Nomenclature and Standards Committee and the Task Force on Chamber Quantification, developed in conjunction with the American College of Cardiology Echocardiography Committee, the American Heart Association, and the European Association of Echocardiography, a branch of the European Society of Cardiology. J Am Soc Echocardiogr 2005;18:1440–63.

11. St John Sutton M, Otterstat JE, Plappert T, et al. Quantitaion of Left Ventricular Volumes and Ejection Fraction in Post-infarction Patients from Biplane and Single Plane Two Dimensional Echocardiograms. A Prospective Longitudinal Study of 1113 Echocardiograms. Eur Heart J 1998;19:808–16.

12. St. John Sutton M, Plappert T. Core lab, no core lab or automated LVEF? Eur J Echocardiogr 2007;8:239–40.

13. Cannesson M, Tanabe M, Suffoletto MS, et al. A novel two-dimensional echocardiographic image analysis system using artificial intelligence-learned pattern recognition for rapid automated ejection fraction. J Am Coll Cardiol 2007;49:217–26.

14. Rahmouni HW, Ky B, Plappert T, et al. Clinical utility of automated assessment of left ventricular ejection fraction using artificial intelligence-assisted border detection. Am Heart J 2008;155:562–70.

15. Mor-Avi V, Sugeng L, Weinert L, et al. Fast measurement of left ventricular mass with real-time three-dimensional echocardiography: comparison with magnetic resonance imaging. Circulation 2004; 110:1814–8.

16. St. John Sutton M, Pfeffer MA, Plappert T, et al. Quantitative two dimensional echocardiographic measurements are major predictors of adverse cardiovascular events following acute myocardial infarction: the protective effects of captopril. Circulation 1994;89:68–75.

17. White HD, Norris RM, Brown MA, et al. Left ventricular end-systolic volume as the major determinant of survival after recovery from myocardial infarction. Circulation 1987;76:44–51.

18. St. John Sutton M, Lee D, Rouleau JL, et al. Left ventricular remodeling and ventricular arrhythmias after myocardial infarction. Circulation 2003;107:2577–82.

19. St John Sutton M, Pfeffer MA, Moye LA, et al. Cardiovascular death and left ventricular remodeling two years after myocardial infarction: baseline predictors and impact of long-term use of captopril. Information from the Survival and Ventricular Enlargement (SAVE) trial. Circulation 1997;96:3294–300.

20. Lamas GA, Vaughan DE, Parisi AF, et al. Effects of left ventricular shape and captopril therapy on exercise capacity after anterior wall acute myocardial infarction. Am J Cardiol 1989;63:1167–73.

21. Pfeffer MA, Braunwald E, Moyé LA, et al. Effect of captopril on mortality and morbidity in patients with left ventricular dysfunction after myocardial infarction. Results of the survival and ventricular enlargement trial. The SAVE Investigators. N Engl J Med 1992;327:669–77.

22. The SOLVD Investigators. Effect of enalapril on mortality and the development of HF in asymptomatic patients with reduced left ventricular ejection fractions. N Engl J Med 1992;327:685–91.

23. Bristow MR, Krause-Steinrauf H, Nuzzo R, et al. Effect of baseline or changes in adrenergic activity on clinical outcomes in the beta-blocker evaluation of survival trial. Circulation 2004;110:1437–42.

24. Abraham WT, Fisher WG, Smith AL, et al. Cardiac resynchronization in chronic HF. N Engl J Med 2002;346:1845–53.

25. Mann DL, Acker MA, Jessup M. Acorn Trial Principal Investigators and Study Coordinators. Clinical evaluation of the CorCap Cardiac Support Device in patients with dilated cardiomyopathy. Ann Thorac Surg 2007;84(4):1226–35.

26. Aurigemma GP, Zile MR, Gaasch WH. Contractile behavior of the left ventricle in diastolic heart failure: with emphasis on regional systolic function. Circulation 2006;113:296–304.

27. Sutherland GR, Stewart MJ, Groundstroem KW, et al. Color Doppler myocardial imaging: a new technique for the assessment of myocardial function. J Am Soc Echocardiogr 1994;7:441–58.

28. Edvardsen T, Skulstad H, Urheim S, et al. Regional myocardial function during acute myocardial ischemia assessed by strain Doppler echocardiography. J Am Coll Cardiol 2001;37:726–30.

29. Abraham TP, Nishimura RA. Myocardial strain: can we finally measure contractility? J Am Coll Cardiol 2001;37:731–4.

30. Gotte MJW, van Rossum AC, Twisk JWR, et al. Quantication of regional contractile function after infarction: strain analysis superior to wall thickening analysis in discriminating infarct from remote myocardium. J Am Coll Cardiol 2001;37:808–17.

31. Korineck J, Wang J, Sengupta PP, et al. Two-dimensional strain-A Doppler independent ultrasound method for quantitation of regional deformation: validation in vitro and in vivo. J Am Soc Echocardiogr 2005;18:1247–53.

32. Artis NJ, Oxborough DL, Williams G, et al. Two-dimensional strain imaging: a new echocardiographic advance with research and clinical applications. Int J Cardiol 2008;123:240–8.

33. Senzaki H, Chen C-H, Kass DA. Singe beat estimation of end-systolic pressure-volume relation in humans: a new method with the potential for non-invasive application. Circulation 1996;94: 2497–506.

34. Grigioni F, Enriquez-Sarano M, Zehr KJ, et al. Regurgitation: long-term outcome and prognostic implications with quantitative Doppler assessment. Circulation 2001;103:1759–64.

35. St John Sutton MG, Plappert T, Abraham WT, et al. Effect of cardiac resynchronization therapy on left ventricular size and function in chronic HF. Circulation 2003;107:1985–90.

36. Linde C, Gold MR, Abraham WT, et al. Randomized trial of cardiac resynchronization in mildly symptomatic HF patients and in asymptomatic patients with left ventricular dysfunction and previous HF symptoms. J Am Coll Cardiol 2008; in press.

37. Cleland JG, Daubert JC, Erdmann E, et al. The effect of cardiac resynchronization on morbidity and mortality in HF. N Engl J Med 2005;352:1539–49.

38. Yu C, Chau E, Sanderson JE, et al. Tissue Doppler echocardiographic evidence of reverse remodeling and improved synchronicity by simultaneously delaying regional contraction after biventricular pacing therapy in HF. Circulation 2002;105:438–45.

39. Chung ES, Leon AR, Tavazzi L, et al. Results of the predictors of response to CRT (PROSPECT) trial. Circulation 2008;117:2608–16.

The Role of Echocardiography in Hemodynamic Assessment in Heart Failure

Jacob Abraham, MD, Theodore P. Abraham, MD*

KEYWORDS

- Heart failure • Hemodynamics • Echocardiography
- Diastolic function • Contractile indices • RV function

Hemodynamic derangement—the inability of the heart to generate adequate cardiac output at normal filling pressures—is a defining feature of the syndrome of heart failure (HF). HF is not a diagnosis but rather is the clinical expression of hemodynamic and neurohormonal abnormalities initiated by a variety of cardiac insults, including myocardial ischemia, cardiomyopathy, valve disease, congenital lesions, and pericardial disease. Careful clinical assessment remains the cornerstone of management of the patient who has HF. The utility of quantitative hemodynamic measurements for routine HF management is unproven, but invasive hemodynamic evaluation still is needed to guide management of HF in specific settings.[1] In such cases, direct measurement of intra-cardiac pressures, vascular resistances, and cardiac output by catheterization remains the reference standard. For routine evaluation and management of HF, however, echocardiography now is recommended as the most useful diagnostic test.[2] Comprehensive Doppler analysis enables accurate assessment of cardiac output, ventricular filling pressures, and vascular resistances (**Table 1**). Echocardiography, however, is not merely a noninvasive surrogate for the right heart catheter. Whereas invasive hemodynamic data represent an instantaneous measurement in time, echocardiography provides details of cardiac structure and function that reflect the consequences of chronic hemodynamic disturbances. Furthermore, echocardiography yields unique information that complements hemodynamic data in assessing the clinical significance of hemodynamic abnormalities and in determining prognosis.

This article reviews the role of echocardiography (M-mode, two-dimensional, spectral, and tissue Doppler) for qualitative and quantitative hemodynamic assessment of the patient who has HF. It highlights the echocardiographic parameters that have the most diagnostic and/or prognostic relevance for patients who have advanced HF. The importance of right heart failure and HF with preserved ejection fraction (HFpEF) is increasingly recognized, and therefore the echocardiographic evaluation of these conditions is emphasized also.

CONTRACTILE FUNCTION OF THE LEFT VENTRICLE

Muscle fiber shortening generates the ventricular stroke volume and thus cardiac output. The extent of muscle shortening, or contractility, is best described by pressure–volume loop analysis, but this method is not feasible in routine clinical practice.[3] Clinical assessment of ventricular contractile performance thus has relied on imperfect and indirect measurements that are sensitive to changes

The Johns Hopkins University, Baltimore, MD, USA

* Corresponding author. Division of Cardiology, The Johns Hopkins University, 600 North Wolfe Street, Baltimore, MD 21287.

E-mail address: tabraha3@jhmi.edu (T.P. Abraham).

Heart Failure Clin 5 (2009) 191–208
doi:10.1016/j.hfc.2008.11.002

heartfailure.theclinics.com

Table 1
Hemodynamic parameters and their echocardiographic correlates

Hemodynamic Parameter	Echocardiographic Correlate	Comment	Reference
Right atrial pressure	IVC diameter and respirophasic variation	Not valid in positive pressure ventilation except to exclude high RAP	41
Pulmonary artery systolic pressure	$4(V_{TR})^2 + RAP$	See **Table 3** for RAP estimation	
Pulmonary artery diastolic pressure	$4(V_{PR})^2 + RAP$	See **Table 3** for RAP estimation	
Pulmonary capillary wedge pressure	E/E_m	$E/E_m > 12$ (TDE of septal mitral annulus) predicts PCWP > 15 mm Hg in patients who have reduced EF	46
Left atrial pressure	$SBP - 4(V_{MR})^2$	Exclude patients with acute MR, prosthetic mitral valve, and LVOT obstruction or peripheral arterial disease of the arm	22
Cardiac output	HR × VTI × area	Accurate measure of LVOT diameter is critical	4
dP/dt	$32/\Delta t$	Δt measured from continuous wave Doppler of MR jet	8
Pulmonary vascular resistance	$10 \times (V_{TR}/RVOT\ VTI) + 0.16$		43

Abbreviation: PCWP, pulmonary capillary wedge pressure.

in loading conditions, such as ventricular volumes, cardiac output, and ejection fraction (EF). Unique echocardiographic indices of myocardial contractile function also have been derived and validated.

Cardiac Output

Quantitation of cardiac output by echocardiography involves Doppler measurement of flow across an orifice. In the absence of an intracardiac shunt or significant valvular regurgitation, the conservation of mass dictates that the volume of blood (Q) flowing through the heart in the steady state is constant. In general, the rate of blood flow can be determined using the hydraulic orifice formula, $dQ/dt = A \times V$, where dQ/dt is flow rate, A is the cross-sectional area of the orifice, and V is the flow velocity. In the cardiovascular system, flow is pulsatile, and thus V varies during the cardiac cycle. Summing (integrating) the flow velocities at each time point during systole yields the stroke distance, or the linear distance blood is pumped during ejection. This measure also is called the velocity–time integral (VTI) because it represents the area under the velocity–time curve.

Stroke volume (SV) then is given as SV = VTI × A and cardiac output (CO) as CO = heart rate (HR) × SV. Pulsed-wave Doppler interrogation of the left ventricular outflow tract (LVOT) at the aortic annulus typically is used for assessment of stroke volume. If continuous-wave Doppler is used, then A must be assessed at the sinotubular junction, the narrowest portion of the aorta, where peak velocity will be recorded. By measuring the LVOT diameter D and assuming a circular cross section, $A = \pi \times (D/2)^2 = \pi\ 0.785 \times D^2$ (**Fig. 1**). An analogous calculation can made for right ventricular (RV) output from the basal short axis. Doppler-based cardiac output measurements correlate well with invasively measured cardiac output, including in critically ill patients.[4]

Accurate quantification of cardiac output using this method requires that several conditions be met. First, precise measurement of the LVOT diameter D is crucial, because any measurement errors are amplified when the term is squared. To avoid this source of error, VTI alone can be used as a surrogate for cardiac output.[5] Second, the diameter and velocity measurements must be made at the same anatomic location and under

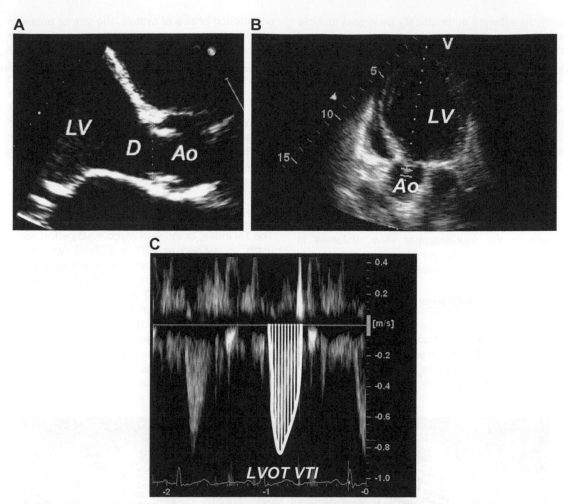

Fig. 1. Measurement of cardiac output using pulse wave Doppler technique. (*A*) Measurement of the LV outflow tract diameter using the edge-to-edge technique. Ao, aorta; D, diameter. (*From* Vivekananthan K, Kalputa T, Mehra M, et al. Usefulness of the combined index of systolic and diastolic myocardial performance to identify cardiac allograft rejection. Am J Cardiol 2002;90(5):518; with permission.) (*B*) Stroke distance (LVOT VTI) is measured using pulse wave Doppler at the aortic annulus. (*C*) VTI measurement of aortic Doppler velocity profile.

similar load and HR conditions. For the latter condition to be met, images must be obtained in close sequence during the echocardiographic examination. Finally, the Doppler beam must be aligned parallel with blood flow to avoid underestimation of the velocity signal.

Ejection Fraction

Although the EF is the most widely used index of contractile function in clinical practice and research, it has major limitations. First, in clinical settings the EF is estimated by visual assessment of endocardial excursion and therefore is susceptible to subjectivity and interobserver variability. Even when cardiac volumes are quantified and the EF is computed, as discussed later, geometric assumptions are made that may be prone to error.

Second, like most indices of contractile function, the EF is sensitive to changes in preload and afterload. Finally, in the management of patients who have HF, there is little correlation between EF and symptoms, exercise capacity, maximum oxygen consumption, or cardiac filling pressures.[6] Despite these limitations, the EF is ingrained in clinical practice because of its proven prognostic ability and relative ease of measurement.

The EF is calculated as EDV − ESV/EDV, where EDV equals end-diastolic volume, and ESV equals end-systolic volume. Calculation of left ventricular (LV) volumes from linear measurements is inaccurate. Professional guidelines recommend that volumes be measured using the biplane method of discs (modified Simpson's rule).[7] With this method, the endocardial border is traced from two orthogonal apical views. Echocardiographic analysis software automatically generates multiple elliptic disks whose cross-sectional area is based on the diameter measured from two- and four-chamber views. The height of each disk is calculated as a fraction of the LV long axis. The volumes of the disks then are summed to provide ventricular volume (**Fig. 2**). If only a single apical view is available, the cross-section of the heart is assumed to be circular; this assumption is most error prone in the setting of regional wall motion abnormalities. If the endocardium is not well visualized, the area–length method is an alternative (**Fig. 3**). This method assumes a bullet-shaped ventricle and requires planimetry of the mid-ventricle short-axis area and the annulus-to-apex length in the four-chamber view. Volumes in systole and diastole are determined from the equation volume = [5(area) (length)]/6.

Rate of Pressure Change During Contraction

The rate of pressure change during contraction (dP/dt), an index of contractility measured at catheterization, also can be estimated noninvasively from the continuous-wave Doppler mitral regurgitation (MR) velocity curve. During the isovolumic

contraction phase of systole, the rate of pressure rise is relatively independent of load. From the Doppler MR spectral signal, the time interval Δt (in milliseconds) between velocities of 1 m/s and 3 m/s on the ascending slope are measured (**Fig. 4**).[8] From the Bernoulli equation ($\Delta P = 4V_{MR}^2$, where ΔP is the LV–LA pressure gradient and V_{MR} is the MR velocity), these MR velocities correspond to a pressure difference of 32 mm Hg (36 − 4 mm Hg), so that $dP/dt = 32/\Delta t$. Using this approach, Doppler-derived dP/dt was found to correlate well with catheter-measured dP/dt.[8]

Tei Index

The Tei index, or index of myocardial performance (IMP), is defined as (IRT + ICT)/ET, where IRT equals isovolumic relaxation time, ICT equals isovolumic contraction time, and ET equals ejection time. The sum IRT + ICT is computed by subtracting ET from the interval between cessation and onset of mitral inflow (**Fig. 5**). This index was proposed as an integrated measure of global systolic and diastolic function. The correlation of IMP with invasively determined indices of ventricular performance, such as dP/dt_{max}, dP/dt_{min},

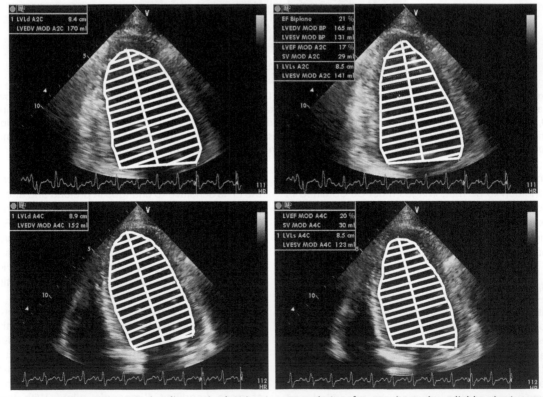

Fig. 2. EF measurement using the disc method. Using image analysis software, the endocardial border is traced manually in systole and diastole in both two- and four-chamber views. The discs technique is applied, yielding EDV and ESV from which EF and SV are computed.

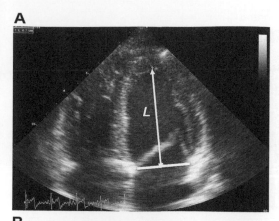

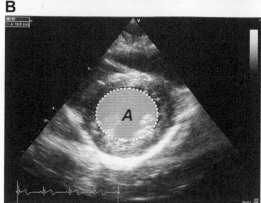

Fig. 3. Area–length method for calculating EF. (*A*) Length L is measured from apex to mitral annulus in the apical four-chamber view. (*B*) Short-axis area *A* is measured at the papillary muscle level. Note that the papillary muscles are excluded from the area calculation.

and tau (τ), is modest.[9] Moreover, in an animal study, IMP was sensitive to acute changes in loading conditions but insensitive to changes in inotropic state.[10] Despite these limitations, IMP retains strong prognostic value in population-based studies. An IMP higher than 0.75 has been shown to predict survival in patients who have dilated cardiomyopathy and severe LV dysfunction.[11]

Strain Rate

Tissue Doppler echocardiography (TDE) quantifies myocardial tissue velocity. Systolic tissue velocity (S_m) correlates modestly with catheter-derived peak dP/dt and has been proposed as a noninvasive index of global contractile function.[12] A significant limitation of TDE is that myocardial velocity is measured relative to an external reference frame (the echocardiography probe) and therefore is affected by tissue translation and tethering.

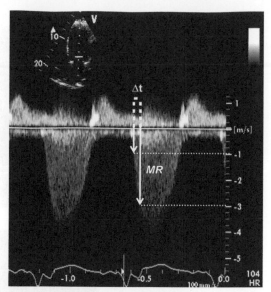

Fig. 4. Use of continuous wave Doppler recording of MR to calculate dP/dt. Time interval (Δt) is measured from 1 m/s to 3 m/s of the velocity curve. dP/dt = 32/Δt.

Strain rate (SR) measurement circumvents this limitation by measuring deformation and velocity relative to a myocardial reference frame. Strain rate, measured in seconds^{-1}, is the spatial derivative of velocity at two points in the myocardium: SR = $V_a - V_b/d$, where $V_a - V_b$ is the instantaneous velocity difference between points *a* and *b* separated by distance *d* (**Fig. 6**). Greenburg and colleagues[13] demonstrated in dogs that peak SR measured at the basal septum by TDE color M-mode cardiography correlated robustly with invasive indices of contractility under varying inotropic conditions. Although promising, clinical application of SR imaging for hemodynamic assessment is limited at present to the detection of reduced contractile function in subclinical cardiomyopathy.[14]

CARDIAC MORPHOLOGY AND REMODELING
Chamber Geometry

Hemodynamic assessment by echocardiography should incorporate cardiac morphology. The heart has limited morphologic responses to pressure and volume overload—hypertrophy and/or dilatation. Chamber geometry provides insight into the nature, chronicity, and severity of adverse loading conditions, and the extent of remodeling is a strong determinant of prognosis. In an echocardiographic substudy of the Beta-blocker Evaluation of Survival Trial (BEST), for example, Grayburn and colleagues[15] found that an LV diastolic volume index (ie, LV diastolic volume/body surface area) greater than 120 mL/m^2 was the only predictor of

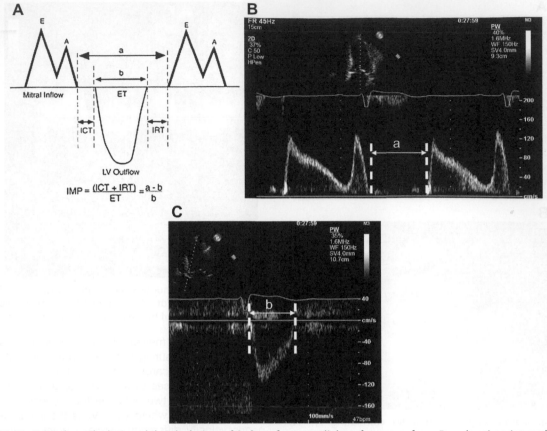

Fig. 5. Tei index calculation. (*A*) Calculation of index of myocardial performance from Doppler time intervals. (*From* Vivekananthan K, Kalputa T, Mehra M, et al. Usefulness of the combined index of systolic and diastolic myocardial performance to identify cardiac allograft rejection. Am J Cardiol 2002;90(5):518; with permission). (*B*) From the apical two-chamber view, the continuous wave Doppler sample volume is placed between the mitral valve leaflet tips to measure the isovolumic contraction time and isovolumic relaxation time, a. (*C*) The ejection time, b, is measured from the outflow ejection time. The Tei index is computed as (a − b)/b.

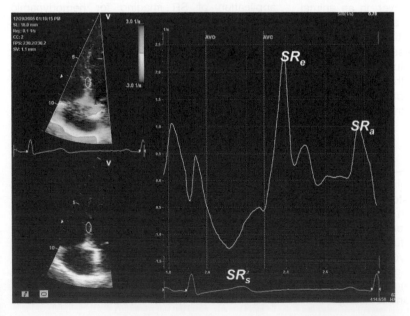

Fig. 6. Strain rate imaging. Strain rate measures the spatial gradient of velocity. Tissue Doppler echocardiography is performed using a high frame rate and narrow sector width (*top panel, left*). A sample volume is placed in the basal septum (*bottom panel, left*). Systolic (SR_s), early diastolic (SR_e), and late diastolic (SR_a) strain rate peaks are shown in the right panel.

death in multivariate analysis. Moreover, once ventricular enlargement is severe (LV diastolic dimension > 7 cm), medical treatment is unlikely to reverse remodeling.[16]

Cardiac remodeling also is central to the pathogenesis of HFpEF. Comparing patients who have HFpEF with a matched control group consisting of individuals who had hypertensive LV hypertrophy but without HF, Melanovsky and colleagues[17] found that LV mass index and maximal left atrial volume (LAV) best distinguished patients from controls. Both groups had similar systolic, diastolic, and vascular dysfunction, suggesting that remodeling was a decisive factor in the transition to HF.

Mitral Regurgitation

Functional MR is a common complication of HF that perpetuates LV remodeling, volume overload, diastolic dysfunction, and secondary pulmonary hypertension (PH). Higher grades of MR are an independent predictor of death in HF.[18] In patients who have dilated cardiomyopathy, poor coaptation of mitral leaflets results from apical displacement of the papillary muscles, abnormalities in regional ventricular wall motion, tethering

of the mitral chordae, annular dilatation, and weakening of mitral closing forces (**Fig. 7**). Although it often is difficult to determine whether MR is a cause or consequence of HF, it is important to distinguish between functional MR and primary valvular diseases (eg, calcification, perforation, flail leaflet, or prolapse), because these lesions dictate different management strategies. Multiple quantitative Doppler methods should be used to quantify the severity of MR, because over-reliance on color Doppler estimation can be misleading.

This caveat is particularly important in acute MR, because the short duration of regurgitation and normal chamber sizes limit jet area and the rapid equilibration of left atrial pressure (LAP) and LV pressure (LVP) reduces jet velocities. Confronted with an acutely ill patient who has pulmonary edema and seemingly mild MR, a careful examination of vena contracta width, pulse Doppler quantification, and Doppler hemodynamic signs of elevated pressures (short aortic regurgitation half-time, pulmonary venous systolic flow reversal, and truncation of MR velocities) may provide the only echocardiographic clues to the true severity of acute MR.

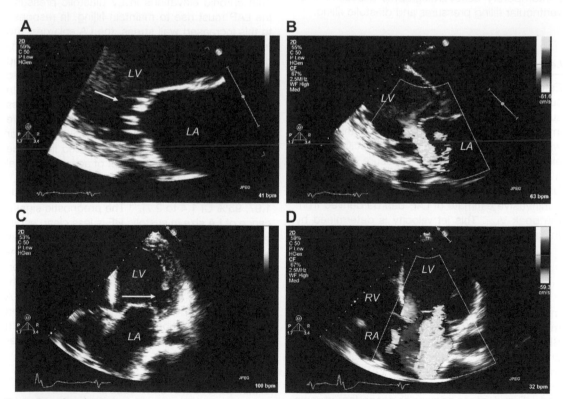

Fig. 7. Functional MR in a 54-year-old man who has non-ischemic dilated cardiomyopathy. (*A*) Tethering of the mitral valve chordae prevents full coaptation of the mitral leaflets in systole. (*B*) Color Doppler demonstrates severe, eccentric MR. (*C*) Apical four-chamber view showing tethering. (*D*) Severe MR with large vena contracta width and jet area.

DIASTOLIC FILLING/FILLING PRESSURES

Diastole encompasses the period of the cardiac cycle from closure of the aortic valve to closure of the mitral valve. During isovolumic relaxation, the LV untwists and de-stiffens. The rate of de-stiffening or relaxation normally is rapid and is characterized by τ or negative dP/dt. The rate of LV filling after mitral valve opening is determined by the instantaneous pressure gradient between LA and LV and the LV compliance (dV/dP). Impaired LV relaxation or reduced LV compliance are fundamental causes of abnormal diastolic filling that can be assessed accurately by echocardiography. Diastolic function also is influenced by a number of other factors, including atrial transport function, ventricular interaction, pericardial constraint, ventricular–vascular coupling (vascular stiffening), and MR.

The severity of diastolic function relates inversely to prognosis in HF (both with preserved and with reduced EF) and directly to symptom severity and B-type natriuretic peptide (BNP) levels.[19–21] A single index of diastolic function analogous to EF remains elusive because of the complex physiology of diastole. Qualitative and quantitative Doppler techniques form the basis of contemporary echocardiographic assessment of ventricular filling pressures and diastolic filling.

Left Atrial Pressure

Estimation of LV and left atrial (LA) diastolic pressures from the pulmonary capillary wedge pressure (PCWP) at right heart catheterization is important in guiding management of the patient who has HF. An insensitive but specific sign of elevated LV end-diastolic pressure (LVEDP) is a "B bump" in the mitral valve M-mode (**Fig. 8**). Using the Bernoulli equation, a quantitative and noninvasive estimate of LAP can be derived from the peak V_{MR}. This jet velocity is determined by the systolic pressure gradient between LV and LA:

$$\Delta P = LV\ systolic\ pressure$$
$$-\ LA\ systolic\ pressure = 4(V_{MR})^2.$$

Brachial artery systolic pressure (SBP) measured by sphygmomanometry is used to estimate LV systolic pressure. Therefore LAP equals SBP $-\ 4(V_{MR})^2$. Applying this method, Gorscan and colleagues[22] studied the correlation between the noninvasive measurement of LAP and simultaneous mean PCWP in 35 stable inpatients who had HF and either primary or secondary chronic MR. This study found a strong correlation between echocardiographic and catheter measurements of LAP, even in the small subgroup (12 patients) who

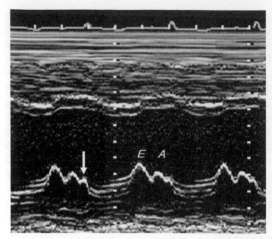

Fig. 8. M-mode cardiography through the mitral leaflets demonstrates a "B hump" (*arrow*) after the *A* excursion, indicating elevated LVEDP.

had phasic *v* waves 10 mm Hg above the mean wedge pressure ($r = 0.87$ versus $r = 0.88$).

Left Atrial Volume

With chronic elevations in LV diastolic pressure, the LAP must rise to maintain filling. In response to this increased wall stress, the LA enlarges and remodels. LAV has been shown to be an independent predictor of atrial fibrillation, stroke, HF, and cardiovascular death and has been proposed to be a marker of chronic diastolic dysfunction.[23] In support of this view, community-based studies have found LA size to be independently predictive of incident HFpEF.[17,24] An LAV of 32 mL/m² or greater was associated with increased incidence of congestive HF, independent of age, myocardial infarction, diabetes mellitus, hypertension, LV hypertrophy, and mitral inflow velocities (HR 1.97, 95% CI 1.4 to 2.7).[24] The prognostic significance of LA size in systolic HF is less clear, especially because diastolic dysfunction is ubiquitous in this population. LAV, rather than linear dimension, is the preferred method of quantification and is computed from the biplane area and length: LAV = $(0.85) \times (A_1) \times (A_2)/L$, where A_1 is the LA area from the four-chamber view, A_2 is LA area from the two-chamber view, and L is the LA length measured from mitral annulus mid-plane to superior LA (**Fig. 9**).

EARLY DIASTOLIC FLOW VELOCITY/LATE DIASTOLIC FLOW VELOCITY

Mitral inflow velocity curves reflect the instantaneous pressure gradient between the LA and LV

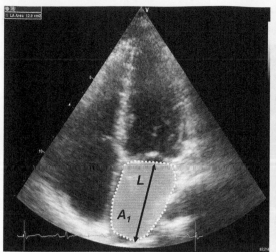 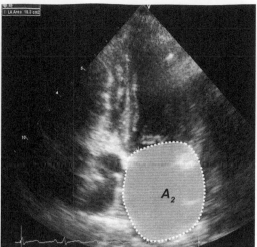

Fig. 9. Area—length method of computing LAV. The length L is chosen as the shorter LA length measured from apical two- or four-chamber. See text for details.

during diastole. Pulse-wave Doppler at the mitral valve leaflet tips records an early diastolic flow velocity (E-wave velocity) followed by a late diastolic flow velocity (A-wave velocity) generated by atrial contraction. In the normal heart, approximately 85% of LV filling occurs during early diastole; therefore, E-wave velocity typically is greater than A-wave velocity. The time interval for the E-wave velocity to decelerate to the zero baseline is the deceleration time (DT) and reflects LV compliance.

Mitral inflow velocities follow a pattern of progression with increasing severity of diastolic abnormalities (**Fig. 10; Table 2**). With mild diastolic dysfunction, LV relaxation is impaired, resulting in reduced E-wave velocity and greater dependence on atrial contraction (higher A-wave velocity) for LV filling, that is, a ratio of E-wave velocity to A-wave velocity (E/A) less than 1. With moderate degrees of diastolic impairment caused by reduced LV compliance, pressures in the LA become elevated. The LA–LV gradient consequently is higher in early diastole, resulting in higher E-wave velocity and a "pseudo-normal" E/A ratio of 1 to 1.5. As LAP increases even further with severe diastolic dysfunction ("restrictive" pattern), the LV fills rapidly and equilibrates with the LA. The E-wave velocity, and therefore the E/A ratio, decreases with age, so that by age 50 years an E/A ratio of less than 1 may be normal. Maneuvers that lower LAP (preload), such as Valsalva's maneuvers, or the use of nitroglycerin, reduce E-wave velocity and thus can convert a restrictive pattern to a pseudo-normal pattern.

In patients who have dilated cardiomyopathy, the presence of a restrictive pattern is associated with poor prognosis, and the inability to convert a restrictive pattern to a pseudo-normal pattern with a Valsalva maneuver portends an even worse outcome.[25] The DT and E/A ratio also can be useful in semiquantitative estimation of LV filling pressures. In a study of patients who had ischemic cardiomyopathy, Giannuzi and colleagues[26] found that a DT of less than120 milliseconds has a high sensitivity and specificity for predicting a PCWP above 20 mm Hg, whereas an E/A ratio greater than 2 had a high specificity (99%) but low sensitivity (43%) for elevated PCWP.

SEMI-QUANTITATIVE ESTIMATION OF FILLING PRESSURES

The mitral E-wave velocity is related directly to LAP and inversely to LV relaxation. In patients who have systolic HF, increased filling pressure (high LAP) and reduced LV relaxation co-exist, so that E-wave velocity alone correlates poorly with mean LAP. Correcting E-wave velocity for abnormal LV relaxation enables accurate estimation of LAP or mean PCWP. The mitral annular velocity (E_m) and the flow propagation velocity (V_p) on color M-mode cardiography have been validated as measures of LV relaxation and have been combined with E-wave velocity to estimate PCWP.

Early diastolic motion of the mitral annulus is influenced by the motion of longitudinally oriented myocardial fibers. The lengthening of these fibers in diastole results in mitral annular descent toward

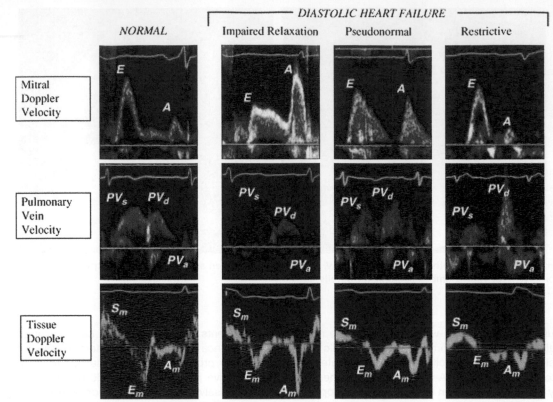

Fig. 10. Changes in Doppler echocardiographic profiles of patients who have different degrees of diastolic heart failure. As diastolic dysfunction worsens, the E/A ratio initially declines; then the stage of pseudo-normalization occurs. As filling pressures continue to rise, a restrictive filling pattern is seen. (*From* Fowler S, Narula J, Gurude-van S. Review of noninvasive imaging for hypertrophic cardiomyopathy syndromes and restrictive physiology. Heart Fail Clin 2006;2(2):218; with permission.)

a relatively fixed apex. The velocity of early mitral annular (E_m) descent reflects LV relaxation and is independent of LAP. Using instrumented dogs, Nagueh and colleagues[27] confirmed that E_m is relatively insensitive to acute alterations in pre-load compared with E-wave velocity. Because E-wave velocity is determined primarily by LAP and LV relaxation, correcting the E-wave velocity for LV relaxation (ie, the E/E_m ratio) allowed accurate assessment of LAP or mean PCWP. An E/E_m

Table 2
Grading of diastolic dysfunction

Pathophysiology	Normal	Grade I ↓ Relaxation	Grade II ↓ Relaxation ↑ LVEDP	Grade III (Reversible) ↓ Relaxation ↓ Compliance ↑ LVEDP	Grade III (Irreversible) ↓ Relaxation ↓↓ Compliance ↑↑ LVEDP
E/A	0.75–1.5	<0.75	0.75–1.5	>1.5	>1.5
DT (ms)	150–200	>200	>200	150–200	<150
IRT (ms)	50–100	>100	50–100	↓	↓
PV_s/PV_d	>1	$PV_s > PV_d$	$PV_s > PV_d$	$PV_s < PV_d$	$PV_s < PV_d$
PV_a (m/s)	<0.35	<0.35	≥0.35	≥0.35	≥0.35
a_{dur}-A_{dur}	<20	<20	≥20	≥20	≥20
E/E_m	<10	<10	≥10	≥10	≥10

ratio (measured at the lateral mitral annulus) greater than 10 detected a PCWP higher than 15 mm Hg with a sensitivity of 97% and specificity of 78%.[27] Similar findings were made using the velocity measured at the septal mitral annulus, with an E/E_m ratio greater than 12 predicting a PCWP greater than 15 mm Hg (**Fig. 11**).[27] The septal annulus now is the preferred site for tissue Doppler imaging, because this location is less influenced by the pericardium.

Ommen and colleagues[28] compared the E/E_m ratio with direct measurement of LVEDP in patients referred for left heart catheterization. An E/E_m ratio less than 8 accurately predicted normal LVEDP, and an E/E_m ratio greater than 15 predicted an elevated LVEDP regardless of EF. E/E_m values between 8 and 15 correlated with a wide range of values of LVEDP, however. Thus, the E/E_m ratio alone is useful in dichotomizing patients as having normal or high LVEDP but cannot classify intermediate values accurately or provide quantitative measurement.

Several caveats are important when the E/E_m ratio is used to estimate filling pressures. First, the E/E_m ratio is insensitive to preload changes in patients who have impaired relaxation but not in patients who have normal relaxation.[29] Moreover, the E/E_m ratio varies with changes in afterload. Borlaug and colleagues[30] demonstrated in humans that E_m is related inversely to arterial load, particularly the late-systolic component caused by arterial wave reflection. The E-wave velocity was not influenced by arterial loading, so the E/E_m ratio varied directly with afterload. These results may explain in part the observation that the E/E_m ratio increases with increasing age.[31] Additionally, the E/E_m ratio does not correlate with PCWP in the setting of severe MR, probably because the regurgitant lesion serves effectively as afterload reduction.[32] A second limitation is that E_m measured at a single point in the heart is assumed to represent global diastolic properties of the heart. Wang and colleagues[33] used two-dimensional speckle tracking to derive a global measure of diastolic strain rate during isovolumic relaxation (SR_{ivr}). Although impractical for routine clinical use, the E/SR_{ivr} ratio accurately predicted PCWP when the E/E_m ratio was indeterminate (ie, in the range from 8–15) and had better accuracy than the E/E_m ratio in patients who had regional wall motion but preserved EF. Finally, in constrictive pericarditis (CP), the E/E_m ratio correlates inversely with PCWP ("annulus paradoxus," as discussed later). Pericardial constriction limits the lateral expansion of the heart during diastole and thereby must increase longitudinal myocardial motion. Because E_m velocity increases in proportion to the severity

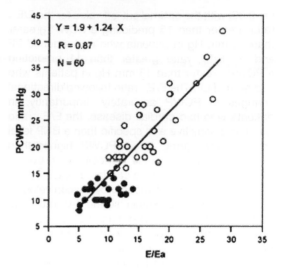

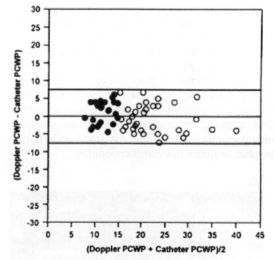

Fig. 11. The upper panel shows the relationship between wedge pressure and E/Ea ratio in 60 patients who had cardiac disease. Ea was measured at the lateral side of the mitral annulus. The lower panel shows the difference between the Doppler estimated and invasively measured mean wedge pressure versus the average of both observations. Solid circles indicate patients who had an impaired relaxation mitral inflow pattern; open circles indicate patients who had pseudo-normal or restrictive LV filling. (*From* Nagueh SF, Middleton KJ, Kopelen HA, et al. Doppler tissue imaging: a noninvasive technique for evaluation of left ventricular relaxation and estimation of filling pressures. J Am Coll Cardiol 1997;30:1531; with permission.)

of constriction, the E/E_m ratio is low despite the increase in LV filling pressure.[34]

Both the E/E_m ratio and BNP levels correlate with LV filling pressures. In patients admitted to an ICU, the E/E_m ratio demonstrated better correlation with PCWP than BNP ($r = 0.69$ versus

$r = 0.32$) with the optimal cut-off value for the E/E_m ratio greater than 15 predicting a PCWP greater than 15 mm Hg in patients who had reduced EF and an E/E_m ratio greater than 11 predicting a PCWP greater than 15 mm Hg in patients who had normal EF. The E/E_m ratio followed directional changes in PCWP accurately. Importantly, in patients who had cardiac disease, the E/E_m ratio was more sensitive and specific than a BNP level greater 400 pg/mL for a PCWP higher than 15 mm Hg, whereas the opposite was true in patients who did not have cardiac disease.[35]

Like E_m, the color M-mode propagation velocity, V_p, is an index of relaxation, so the E/V_p ratio also tracks with PCWP. V_p is obtained by placing the color M-mode cursor in the direction of mitral inflow as seen by color Doppler. The slope of the line along the edge of the first aliasing velocity in early diastole is the propagation velocity (normal > 50 cm/s) (**Fig. 12**). Garcia and colleagues[36] studied a heterogeneous patient group in a cardiac ICU and related PCWP to the E/V_p ratio. They found that a E/V_p ratio greater than 2 correlated with a PCWP greater than 15 mm Hg. In contemporary practice, E_m is used more commonly because it generally is easier to obtain and interpret than V_p. In addition, V_p can be artificially elevated when the LV cavity is small, as in hypertrophic or restrictive cardiomyopathy.

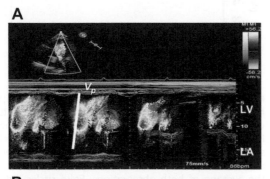

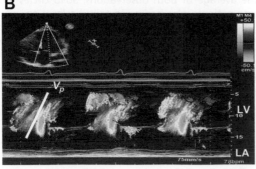

Fig. 12. V_p (*A*) in a normal subject and (*B*) in a patient who has cardiomyopathy. V_p is measured as the slope of the line along the first aliasing velocity, as indicated.

Pulmonary Venous Inflow

LA filling from the pulmonary veins provides additional insight into LV filling pressures. The normal pulmonary venous inflow velocity curve is characterized by inflow biphasic peaks in systole (PV_s) and diastole (PV_d) followed by a small atrial flow reversal (PV_a) whose duration is a_{dur} (see **Fig. 10**). The two systolic peaks can be resolved only by transesophageal echocardiography and correspond to LA relaxation and mitral annular descent toward the apex. PV_d, the velocity of diastolic flow into the LA, reflects the transmitral filling pressure gradient. With mitral valve opening, the LA and LV operate effectively as a single receiving chamber for pulmonary venous inflow, and therefore PV_d is influenced by the same determinants as E-wave velocity. Atrial contraction results in blood flow across the mitral valve as well as backward into the pulmonary veins. PV_a is determined by the interplay between compliance properties of the LA and LV and by atrial contractile function. In the normal heart with low LAP (ie, $PV_s/PV_d \geq 1$), PV_a is low (< 0.35 m/s), and a_{dur} is short. With increasing LAP pressure and reduced LV compliance, systolic flow into the LA decreases, PV_d exceeds PV_s and PV_a is greater than 0.35 m/s. In addition, a_{dur} is prolonged because of the increased flow reversal into the pulmonary veins. An a_{dur} 20 milliseconds greater than the duration of the mitral A wave (A_{dur}) was found to predict an LVEDP greater than 15 mm Hg with moderate sensitivity and specificity.[37]

Interrogation of pulmonary venous inflow is challenging in actual practice. From a transthoracic apical view, a sample volume is placed 1 to 2 cm inside the right superior pulmonary vein. At this depth, signal strength is limited, and it can be difficult to place the sample volume accurately.

PULMONARY CIRCULATION AND RIGHT HEART FUNCTION

RV dysfunction and secondary PH are critical determinants of functional capacity and survival in HF. Although PH in HF is caused primarily by pulmonary venous hypertension, there is little relationship between the degree of LV dysfunction and pulmonary artery pressure (PAP) because of the variable degree of diastolic impairment, MR, and LA size and compliance. Echocardiographic predictors of PH are a restrictive mitral inflow pattern and the severity of MR.[38]

RV function is an independent and additive prognosticator in PH complicating HF. The importance of RV function was illustrated by Ghio and colleagues,[39] who found that patients who had RV dysfunction and normal PAP had a prognosis similar to those who had normal RV function and PH, whereas those who had RV dysfunction and PH had considerably worse outcomes.

The complex geometry of the RV and suboptimal endocardial border definition preclude a reliable tomographic assessment of ventricular volumes and function. Because of the orientation of muscle fibers in the RV, contraction occurs predominantly along the longitudinal plane. Consequently, displacement of the tricuspid annulus toward the RV apex (tricuspid annular plane systolic excursion, TAPSE) is a reliable, easily measured surrogate for RV EF. In a population of patients who had advanced HF, Ghio and colleagues[40] showed that a TAPSE greater than 14 mm provided incremental prognostic information to functional class, LV function, and diastolic function and was measured more reliably than RV fractional area change or RV axis shortening. TAPSE is obtained by placing the M-mode cursor through the lateral tricuspid annulus and measuring the systolic motion of the annulus (**Fig. 13**).

Measures of RV diastolic function are analogous to those of the LV and are useful in characterizing various hemodynamic states. Unlike mitral inflow velocities, early and late tricuspid inflow peak velocities vary with respiration, increasing with inspiration because of increased systemic venous return and decreasing with expiration. Both superior vena cava and hepatic venous inflow patterns reflect the mechanics of RA filling and are characterized by systolic forward flow, diastolic forward flow, systolic flow reversal, and diastolic flow reversal (**Fig. 14**). These patterns of RA filling correlate with the jugular venous pressure curve.

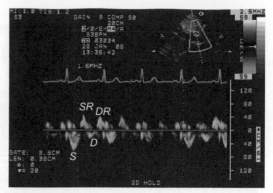

Fig. 14. Pulse Doppler evaluation of the hepatic veins demonstrates systolic (S) and diastolic (D) forward-filling velocities and flow reversal in systole (SR) and diastole (DR).

In normal subjects, the systolic forward flow is greater than the diastolic forward flow, and the systolic flow reversal and the diastolic flow reversal are low. With increasing RA pressure, the systolic forward flow decreases, and the diastolic forward flow increases, so that the diastolic forward flow is greater than the systolic forward flow; with severely increased RA pressure, the systolic flow reversal and the diastolic flow reversal become prominent. In patients who have cardiomyopathy both systolic flow reversal and diastolic flow reversal increase with inspiration. Tricuspid regurgitation (TR) results in a prominent S velocity.

Right ventricular systolic pressure (RVSP), which equals pulmonary artery systolic pressure (PASP) in the absence of RV outflow tract (RVOT) obstruction, is calculated reliably using the simplified Bernoulli equation from the velocity of the TR jet (V_{TR}) and RA pressure (RAP) (**Fig. 15**): RVSP = PASP = $4(V_{TR})^2$ + RAP. The RAP is estimated from bedside examination of the jugular venous pressure or is inferred from the inferior vena cava (IVC) dimension and the response to the "sniff" test (**Table 3**).[41] The normal IVC measures 15 to 25 mm and decreases by more than 50% with quiet inspiration. The absence of inspiratory IVC narrowing by more than 50% of the expiratory dimension suggests a RAP greater than 10 mm Hg, and distension of the IVC by more than 25 mm with lack of respiratory variation indicates an RAP of 20 mm Hg. These correlations are not accurate in ventilated patients because of positive-pressure ventilation, but a small IVC that collapses with respiration effectively excludes an elevated RAP. Other two-dimensional echocardiography findings that correlate with elevated RAP include leftward bowing of the interatrial septum, dilatation of the

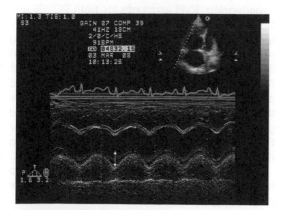

Fig. 13. Measurement of TAPSE in a patient who has pulmonary arterial hypertension. The M-mode cursor is placed through the lateral tricuspid annulus.

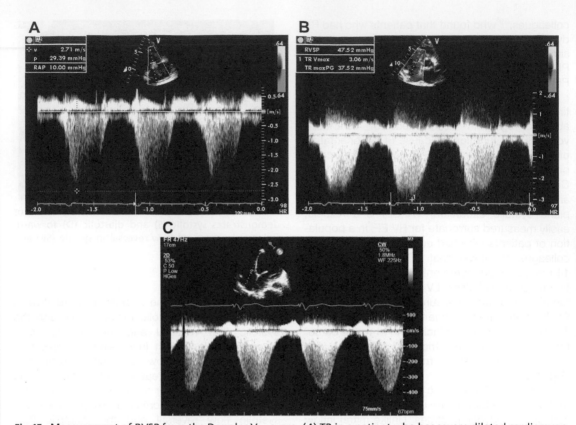

Fig. 15. Measurement of RVSP from the Doppler V_{TR} curve. (A) TR in a patient who has severe dilated cardiomyopathy. Note the signal drop-out in the second half of systole. Peak V_{TR} is 2.7 m/s, and RVSP is 30 mm Hg. (B) Doppler interrogation from the basal short-axis view in the same patient. The TR signal intensity is much stronger because of better alignment of the Doppler beam with the regurgitant jet. The peak V_{TR} is 3.0 m/s, and RVSP is 38 mm Hg. (C) TR Doppler curve from another patient who has heart failure. The V_{TR} is 4 m/s, and RVSP is 75 mm Hg.

coronary sinus, right-to-left shunting through a patent foramen ovale, and enlargement of the RA.

To avoid underestimation of RVSP, it is important to measure the peak V_{TR} using continuous-wave Doppler from a parallel intercept angle, usually from an apical four-chamber or RV inflow view. Agitated saline can be used to improve suboptimal Doppler signals. Overestimation will occur if the MR jet is confused for the TR jet, because V_{MR} usually is high, because of the greater pressure gradient between LV and LA. PH is diagnosed when the RVSP exceeds 35 mm Hg. In a large number of normal subjects RVSP has been found to increase with age and obesity, indicating that the normal range of RVSP may be as high as 40 mm Hg.[42] Applying a similar approach enables estimation of the pulmonary artery diastolic pressure (PADP) from the pulmonary regurgitant jet velocity (V_{PR}): PADP = $4(V_{PR})^2$ + RAP.

The PAP is a surrogate for pulmonary vascular resistance (PVR). An abnormal PAP, whether derived from echocardiography or invasive measurement, is not synonymous with pulmonary vascular disease, however. The PAP may be elevated despite normal pulmonary vasculature because of increased flow through the pulmonary circulation, as occurs with left-to-right shunts, or passively elevated because of pulmonary venous hypertension. PVR accounts for both PCWP and CO and therefore is used in determining candidacy for heart transplantation and in assessing response to vasodilator therapy in HF. The PVR is calculated from catheter measurements: PVR = mean PAP − PCWP/CO. Abbas and colleagues[43] used echocardiography to assess the PVR noninvasively. These authors found good correlation (r = 0.93) between the V_{TR}/RVOT VTI ratio and catheter-based PVR using the equation PVR = 10 × (V_{TR}/RVOT VTI) + 0.16.

At a cut-off value of 0.2, the V_{TR}/RVOT VTI ratio had a sensitivity of 70% and specificity of 94% for determining a PVR greater than 2 Woods units.

Qualitative evidence of chronic RV pressure or volume overload includes RV chamber dilatation and hypertrophy. Acute RV dilatation and

Table 3
Estimation of right atrial pressure

IVC Diameter (cm)	Respiratory Variation	Estimated RAP (mm Hg)
Small (<1.5)	Collapse	0–5
Normal (1.5–2.5)	Decrease by >50%	5–10
Normal	Decrease by <50%	10–15
Dilated (>2.5)	Decrease by <50%	15–20
Dilated	No change	>20

hypocontractility can occur with acute pressure overload caused by major pulmonary embolism and may be distinguished from chronic RV disease by preserved RV apical contractility ("McConnell's sign") and the absence of RV hypertrophy.[44] The pattern of septal motion also provides insight into the hemodynamic state of the RV (**Fig. 16**). In RV volume overload, the leftward bowing of the interventricular septum occurs in diastole with normal systolic curvature, whereas pressure overload causes septal flattening in both systole and early diastole.[45]

CONSTRICTION VERSUS RESTRICTION

CP and restrictive cardiomyopathy (RCM) must be considered in any patient who has symptoms and signs of HF and normal systolic function. The clinical distinction between these two entities can be difficult, but in most cases echocardiography can aid in the diagnosis. Two-dimensional echocardiography findings characteristic of infiltrative restrictive cardiomyopathy include significant TR and MR, marked bi-atrial enlargement, and normal systolic function. A myocardium that is thickened

and has a "sparkling" appearance on echocardiogram suggests amyloidosis, although the absence of these findings does not exclude amyloid or other infiltrative cardiomyopathy. Atrial enlargement typically is less prominent in CP. M-mode and two-dimensional findings suggestive of CP include a thickened pericardium, exaggerated septal motion, dilated IVC, and diastolic flattening of the LV posterior wall (**Fig. 17**). None of these findings are sensitive or specific.

The utility of echocardiography in distinguishing CP from RCM therefore rests primarily on its ability to demonstrate noninvasively the hallmark mechanisms of CP: (1) the dissociation of intracardiac and intrathoracic pressures and (2) exaggerated ventricular interdependence in diastolic filling. Because the rigid pericardium does not effectively transmit respiratory changes in intrathoracic pressure to the heart, the transmitral filling gradient (PCWP–LVP) tracks respiratory changes in the PCWP, decreasing with inspiration and increasing with expiration. Reciprocal respiratory changes occur in the RV filling gradient. Consequently, inspiration decreases the mitral E-wave and increases the tricuspid E-wave and hepatic vein

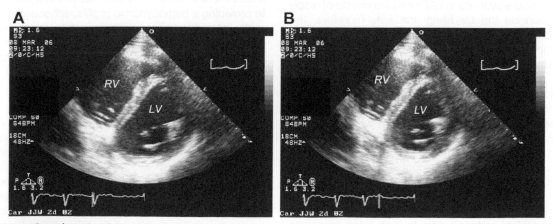

Fig. 16. Septal motion in a patient who has RV pressure and volume overload. (*A*) At end-diastole, the septum is mid-line, and the LV has a D-shape. (*B*) At end-systole, the septum remains mid-line because RV and LV pressures are equal.

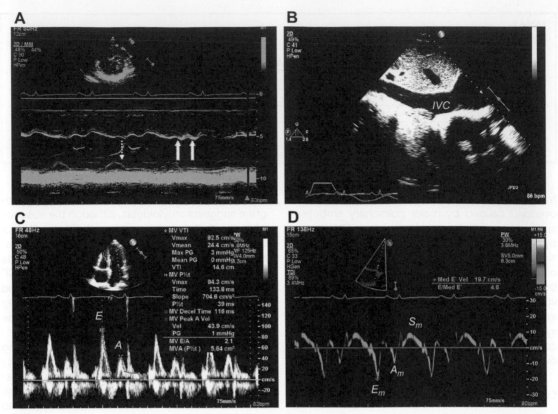

Fig. 17. Echocardiographic findings in constrictive pericarditis. (*A*) M-mode images show abnormal septal motion (*solid arrows*) and flattening of the posterior (*dashed arrow*) during early diastole. (*B*) The dilated IVC indicates elevated right atrial pressure. (*C*) Restrictive mitral inflow pattern with rapid deceleration time (116 ms). (*D*) Myocardial velocity at the basal medial septum is very high (E_m= 19.7 cm/s). The E/E_m is low (4.9) despite elevated filling pressures (annulus paradoxus). At subsequent right heart catheterization, the pulmonary capillary wedge pressure was 24 mm Hg.

diastolic velocity, whereas expiration produces opposite changes and increases diastolic flow reversal in the hepatic veins. Traditionally, a 25% variation in the peak E-wave velocity is used as the threshold value. An important caveat is that marked elevations in LAP blunt the effects of respiration on the LV filling gradient. Therefore, the absence of respiratory variation in E-wave velocity should not exclude the diagnosis of CP, especially when other features of CP are present.

Tissue Doppler of the mitral annulus is useful in differentiating CP from RCM. In myocardial disease, E_m is reduced (< 7 cm/s) because of abnormal myocardial relaxation, whereas in CP, E_m is normal or elevated. Pericardial constraint limits the lateral expansion of the heart, and longitudinal lengthening becomes exaggerated. As filling pressure increases in CP, E_m increases linearly, exactly the opposite of its behavior in myocardial disease. Consequently, the E/E_m ratio is normal or reduced despite high filling pressures in CP (annulus paradoxus) but is low in myocardial disease (see **Fig. 17**).

SUMMARY

Qualitative and quantitative hemodynamic data can be obtained through echocardiography, making it a valuable noninvasive tool in the routine assessment of the patient who has HF. In addition to providing a hemodynamic profile, echocardiography provides unique and powerful prognostic data that cannot be obtained by catheterization. Thus, echocardiography is the diagnostic test of choice in the initial hemodynamic evaluation of HF.

REFERENCES

1. Stevenson LW. Are hemodynamic goals viable in tailoring heart failure therapy? Hemodynamic goals are relevant. Circulation 2006;113(7):1020–7 [discussion 1033].
2. Hunt SA. ACC/AHA 2005 guideline update for the diagnosis and management of chronic heart failure in the adult: a report of the American College of Cardiology/American Heart Association Task Force on Practice Guidelines (Writing Committee to Update the 2001 Guidelines for the Evaluation and

Management of Heart Failure). J Am Coll Cardiol 2005;46(6):e1–e82.

3. Kass DA, Maughan WL, Guo ZM, et al. Comparative influence of load versus inotropic states on indexes of ventricular contractility: experimental and theoretical analysis based on pressure-volume relationships. Circulation 1987;76(6):1422–36.

4. Nishimura RA, Callahan MJ, Schaff HV, et al. Noninvasive measurement of cardiac output by continuous-wave Doppler echocardiography: initial experience and review of the literature. Mayo Clin Proc 1984; 59(7):484–9.

5. Goldman JH, Schiller NB, Lim DC, et al. Usefulness of stroke distance by echocardiography as a surrogate marker of cardiac output that is independent of gender and size in a normal population. Am J Cardiol 2001;87(4):499–502, A8.

6. Lapu-Bula R, Robert A, De Kock M, et al. Relation of exercise capacity to left ventricular systolic function and diastolic filling in idiopathic or ischemic dilated cardiomyopathy. Am J Cardiol 1999;83(5): 728–34.

7. Lang RM, Bierig M, Devereux RB, et al. Recommendations for chamber quantification: a report from the American Society of Echocardiography's Guidelines and Standards Committee and the Chamber Quantification Writing Group, developed in conjunction with the European Association of Echocardiography, a branch of the European Society of Cardiology. J Am Soc Echocardiogr 2005;18(12):1440–63.

8. Bargiggia GS, Bertucci C, Recusani F, et al. A new method for estimating left ventricular dP/dt by continuous wave Doppler-echocardiography. Validation studies at cardiac catheterization. Circulation 1989;80(5):1287–92.

9. Tei C, Nishimura RA, Seward JB, et al. Noninvasive Doppler-derived myocardial performance index: correlation with simultaneous measurements of cardiac catheterization measurements. J Am Soc Echocardiogr 1997;10(2):169–78.

10. Cheung MM, Smallhorn JF, Redington AN, et al. The effects of changes in loading conditions and modulation of inotropic state on the myocardial performance index: comparison with conductance catheter measurements. Eur Heart J 2004;25(24): 2238–42.

11. Peltier M, Slama M, Garbi S, et al. Prognostic value of Doppler-derived myocardial performance index in patients with left ventricular systolic dysfunction. Am J Cardiol 2002;90(11):1261–3.

12. Yamada H, Oki T, Tabata T, et al. Assessment of left ventricular systolic wall motion velocity with pulsed tissue Doppler imaging: comparison with peak dP/dt of the left ventricular pressure curve. J Am Soc Echocardiogr 1998;11(5):442–9.

13. Greenberg NL, Firstenberg MS, Castro PL, et al. Doppler-derived myocardial systolic strain rate is a strong index of left ventricular contractility. Circulation 2002;105(1):99–105.

14. Koyama J, Ray-Sequin PA, Falk RH. Longitudinal myocardial function assessed by tissue velocity, strain, and strain rate tissue Doppler echocardiography in patients with AL (primary) cardiac amyloidosis. Circulation 2003;107(19):2446–52.

15. Grayburn PA, Appleton CP, DeMaria AN, et al. Echocardiographic predictors of morbidity and mortality in patients with advanced heart failure: the Beta-blocker Evaluation of Survival Trial (BEST). J Am Coll Cardiol 2005;45(7):1064–71.

16. Levine TB, Levine AB, Bolenbaugh J, et al. Impact of left ventricular size on pharmacologic reverse remodeling in heart failure. Clin Cardiol 2000;23(5): 355–8.

17. Melenovsky V, Borlaug BA, Rosen B, et al. Cardiovascular features of heart failure with preserved ejection fraction versus nonfailing hypertensive left ventricular hypertrophy in the urban Baltimore community: the role of atrial remodeling/dysfunction. J Am Coll Cardiol 2007;49(2):198–207.

18. Trichon BH, Felker GM, Shaw LK, et al. Relation of frequency and severity of mitral regurgitation to survival among patients with left ventricular systolic dysfunction and heart failure. Am J Cardiol 2003; 91(5):538–43.

19. Bursi F, Weston SA, Redfield MM, et al. Systolic and diastolic heart failure in the community. JAMA 2006; 296(18):2209–16.

20. Packer M. Abnormalities of diastolic function as a potential cause of exercise intolerance in chronic heart failure. Circulation 1990;81(2 Suppl):III78–86.

21. Persson H, Lonn E, Edner M, et al. Diastolic dysfunction in heart failure with preserved systolic function: need for objective evidence: results from the CHARM Echocardiographic Substudy-CHARMES. J Am Coll Cardiol 2007;49(6):687–94.

22. Gorcsan Jr, Snow FR, Paulsen W, et al. Noninvasive estimation of left atrial pressure in patients with congestive heart failure and mitral regurgitation by Doppler echocardiography. Am Heart J 1991; 121(3 Pt 1):858–63.

23. Abhayaratna WP, Seward JB, Appleton CP, et al. Left atrial size: physiologic determinants and clinical applications. J Am Coll Cardiol 2006;47(12): 2357–63.

24. Takemoto Y, Barnes ME, Seward JB, et al. Usefulness of left atrial volume in predicting first congestive heart failure in patients > or = 65 years of age with well-preserved left ventricular systolic function. Am J Cardiol 2005;96(6):832–6.

25. Pinamonti B, Di Lenarda A, Sinagra G, et al. Restrictive left ventricular filling pattern in dilated cardiomyopathy assessed by Doppler echocardiography: clinical, echocardiographic and hemodynamic correlations and prognostic implications. Heart

Muscle Disease Study Group. J Am Coll Cardiol 1993;22(3):808–15.

26. Giannuzzi P, Imparato A, Temporelli PL, et al. Doppler-derived mitral deceleration time of early filling as a strong predictor of pulmonary capillary wedge pressure in postinfarction patients with left ventricular systolic dysfunction. J Am Coll Cardiol 1994;23(7):1630–7.

27. Nagueh SF, Sun H, Kopelen HA, et al. Hemodynamic determinants of the mitral annulus diastolic velocities by tissue Doppler. J Am Coll Cardiol 2001;37(1):278–85.

28. Ommen SR, Nishimura RA, Appleton CP, et al. Clinical utility of Doppler echocardiography and tissue Doppler imaging in the estimation of left ventricular filling pressures: a comparative simultaneous Doppler-catheterization study. Circulation 2000; 102(15):1788–94.

29. Firstenberg MS, Levine BD, Garcia MJ, et al. Relationship of echocardiographic indices to pulmonary capillary wedge pressures in healthy volunteers. J Am Coll Cardiol 2000;36(5):1664–9.

30. Borlaug BA, Melenovsky V, Redfield MM, et al. Impact of arterial load and loading sequence on left ventricular tissue velocities in humans. J Am Coll Cardiol 2007;50(16):1570–7.

31. De Sutter J, De Backer J, Van de Veire N, et al. Effects of age, gender, and left ventricular mass on septal mitral annulus velocity (E') and the ratio of transmitral early peak velocity to E' (E/E'). Am J Cardiol 2005;95(8):1020–3.

32. Olson JJ, Costa SP, Young CE, et al. Early mitral filling/diastolic mitral annular velocity ratio is not a reliable predictor of left ventricular filling pressure in the setting of severe mitral regurgitation. J Am Soc Echocardiogr 2006;19(1):83–7.

33. Wang J, Khoury DS, Thohan V, et al. Global diastolic strain rate for the assessment of left ventricular relaxation and filling pressures. Circulation 2007; 115(11):1376–83.

34. Ha JW, Oh JK, Ling LH, et al. Annulus paradoxus: transmitral flow velocity to mitral annular velocity ratio is inversely proportional to pulmonary capillary wedge pressure in patients with constrictive pericarditis. Circulation 2001;104(9):976–8.

35. Dokainish H, Zoghbi WA, Lakkis NM, et al. Optimal noninvasive assessment of left ventricular filling pressures: a comparison of tissue Doppler echocardiography and B-type natriuretic peptide in patients with pulmonary artery catheters. Circulation 2004; 109(20):2432–9.

36. Garcia MJ, Ares MA, Asher C, et al. An index of early left ventricular filling that combined with pulsed Doppler peak E velocity may estimate capillary wedge pressure. J Am Coll Cardiol 1997;29(2):448–54.

37. Rossvoll O, Hatle LK. Pulmonary venous flow velocities recorded by transthoracic Doppler ultrasound: relation to left ventricular diastolic pressures. J Am Coll Cardiol 1993;21(7):1687–96.

38. Enriquez-Sarano M, Rossi A, Seward JB, et al. Determinants of pulmonary hypertension in left ventricular dysfunction. J Am Coll Cardiol 1997;29(1):153–9.

39. Ghio S, Gavazzi A, Campana C, et al. Independent and additive prognostic value of right ventricular systolic function and pulmonary artery pressure in patients with chronic heart failure. J Am Coll Cardiol 2001;37(1):183–8.

40. Ghio S, Recusani F, Klersy C, et al. Prognostic usefulness of the tricuspid annular plane systolic excursion in patients with congestive heart failure secondary to idiopathic or ischemic dilated cardiomyopathy. Am J Cardiol 2000;85(7):837–42.

41. Kircher BJ, Himelman RB, Schiller NB. Noninvasive estimation of right atrial pressure from the inspiratory collapse of the inferior vena cava. Am J Cardiol 1990;66(4):493–6.

42. McQuillan BM, Picard MH, Leavitt M, et al. Clinical correlates and reference intervals for pulmonary artery systolic pressure among echocardiographically normal subjects. Circulation 2001;104(23):2797–802.

43. Abbas AE, Fortuin FD, Schiller NB, et al. A simple method for noninvasive estimation of pulmonary vascular resistance. J Am Coll Cardiol 2003;41(6): 1021–7.

44. McConnell MV, Solomon SD, Rayan ME, et al. Regional right ventricular dysfunction detected by echocardiography in acute pulmonary embolism. Am J Cardiol 1996;78(4):469–73.

45. Louie EK, Rich S, Levitsky S, et al. Doppler echocardiographic demonstration of the differential effects of right ventricular pressure and volume overload on left ventricular geometry and filling. J Am Coll Cardiol 1992;19(1):84–90.

46. Nagueh SF, Middleton KJ, Kopelen HA, et al. Doppler tissue imaging: a noninvasive technique for evaluation of left ventricular relaxation and estimation of filling pressures. J Am Coll Cardiol 1997; 30(6):1527–33.

Noninvasive Measurement of Cardiac Output During Exercise by Inert Gas Rebreathing Technique

Gaia Cattadori, MD[a], Jean-Paul Schmid, MD[a,b],
Piergiuseppe Agostoni, MD, PhD[a,c],*

KEYWORDS

- Cardiac output • Exercise • Heart failure • Inert gases

This article focuses on the physiologic basis of oxygen delivery and peak oxygen consumption and highlights the potential advantage of a noninvasive cardiac output measurement during exercise. We focus on the use of noninvasive cardiac output (CO) determination as a tool to implement oxygen consumption (VO_2) measurement during exercise in patients with chronic heart failure (CHF) in stable clinical conditions. Although the VO_2 versus CO relationship during exercise in normal subjects is linear and has a predictable slope so that exercise CO can be estimated from VO_2 in normal subjects,[1] this is not the case in patients who have heart failure, in whom the simultaneous measurement of VO_2 and CO becomes necessary.

PHYSIOLOGY OF OXYGEN CONSUMPTION AND DETERMINANTS DURING EXERCISE

Respiratory gas analysis offers the gold standard of exercise capacity measurements. The most frequently reported parameter is peak VO_2, which corresponds to CO times the arteriovenous oxygen difference ($C(a-v)O_2$). $C(a-v)O_2$ is the differences between arterial (CaO_2) and venous (CvO_2) oxygen content. CvO_2 is caused by the mixture

of blood arriving from two physiologically distinct sources: veins draining blood from exercising muscles and the heart, where gas changes during exercise occurs, and veins arriving from organs, the activity of which is not influenced by exercise. In normal subjects during exercise, blood flow to working muscles progressively increases and blood flow to organs not directly involved in exercise remains constant. Conversely, during exercise in patients who have CHF, a redistribution of blood flow takes place so that while blood flow to working muscles increases, blood flow to organs not directly involved in exercise reduces. This allows a greater blood flow increase toward exercising muscles even when CO increase is blunted. The redistribution of blood means an increase in oxygen extraction even in organs not directly involved in exercise.

Oxygen content in the blood depends on three factors: hemoglobin concentration, PO_2, and oxy/hemoglobin dissociation curve. In the systemic artery, oxygen content increases during exercise, mainly above the anaerobic threshold, because of an increase in hemoglobin. At rest, the oxygen/hemoglobin saturation curve is already on its flat portion, so that the PO_2 increase

[a] Università di Milano, Milan, Italy
[b] Bern University Hospital and University of Bern, Bern, Switzerland
[c] University of Washington, Seattle, WA, USA
* Corresponding author. Centro Cardiologico Monzino, IRCCS, Istituto di Cardiologia, Università di Milano, via Parea 4, 20138 Milan, Italy.
E-mail address: piergiuseppe.agostoni@ccfm.it (P. Agostoni).

Heart Failure Clin 5 (2009) 209–215
doi:10.1016/j.hfc.2008.11.004
1551-7136/08/$ – see front matter © 2009 Elsevier Inc. All rights reserved.

observed during exercise in normal patients and patients who have CHF does not significantly affect oxygen content.[2] Exercise-induced hemo-concentration is caused by an oncotic effect of the increased intracellular lactate, but a role played by spleen contraction cannot be excluded.[3] Reduction of spleen size has been documented after exercise in healthy humans. In patients who have thalassemia who have under-gone splenectomy, exercise-induced hemocon-centration is lower compared with patients who did not undergo splenectomy.[4] Hemoconcentra-tion accounts for approximately 20% of the increase in $C(a-v)O_2$ at peak exercise.[2]

In the pulmonary artery, oxygen content reduces progressively throughout the entire exer-cise, which before reaching anaerobic threshold is caused by a reduction in PO_2 and—above anaerobic threshold—a shift in the oxy/hemo-globin dissociation curve (the "so-called" Bohr effect) and a reduction of PO_2.[5] In the femoral vein, which drains blood from active muscles, the reduction of oxygen content is caused by PO_2 changes before the anaerobic threshold and the Bohr effect afterwards. PO_2 reduces up to the anaerobic threshold, whereas oxyhemoglobin saturation reduces throughout the entire test.[2,5] PO_2 reduction and the Bohr effect account for 60% and 20%, respectively, of $C(a-v)O_2$ increase at peak exercise.[2]

In patients who have CHF, at anaerobic threshold $C(a-v)O_2$ is a function of heart failure severity with little differences among subjects with the same heart failure severity (**Table 1**). Accordingly, in patients who have CHF, only at the anaerobic threshold is it possible to estimate CO if VO_2 is known.[6] On the other hand, in normal subjects, $C(a-v)O_2$ increases linearly with progres-sion of workload,[1] and VO_2 mainly reflects CO throughout the entire exercise.

WHY PEAK OXYGEN CONSUMPTION IS NOT ENOUGH

VO_2 at peak exercise is the most frequently used parameter to assess exercise capacity in patients who have CHF. To account for differences in peak VO_2 related to age, sex, weight, and height, several VO_2 normalization procedures have been reported, the most frequently used being peak VO_2/body weight. This normalization does not take into account age, sex, a subject's fitness, and obesity, however. Patient fitness is an important determinant of exercise capacity, but fitness has a limited relevance in cardiac perfor-mance and an important relevance in muscle performance. Although normalized for body

weight, the VO_2/kg value does not respect the fact that fat has a low VO_2, and in cases of obesity, VO_2/kg underestimates the true VO_2. This is a rele-vant issue because obesity is a comorbid factor frequently observed in patients who have CHF, and based on a misleading low VO_2/kg value, heart failure is frequently wrongly diagnosed in obese subjects.

Peak VO_2 is enough to define prognosis in patients who have CHF if peak VO_2 is more than 18 mL/min/kg or less than 10 mL/min/kg, but in the latter case, anaerobic threshold needs to be achieved.[7] Data are less clear if peak VO_2 is between 10 and 18 mL/min/kg, however, which is the case for most patients who have CHF. Several groups have found no statistical difference in survival between patients who have CHF with peak VO_2 between 10 and 14 mL/min/kg and patients with peak VO_2 between 14 and 18 mL/min/kg. Peak exercise VO_2 can be influenced by several noncardiac factors, such as muscle de-conditioning, motivation, anemia, abnormal reflex response, and obesity. Few therapeutic options (eg, beta-blockers, cardiac resynchronization therapy) that improve the quality of life, survival, and hospitalization rates are not associated with significant changes in peak VO_2. Accordingly, Wasserman and colleagues[8] recently demon-strated that if a patient who has CHF has a peak VO_2 of more than 12 mL/min/kg, CRT does not increase functional capacity and likely remains a useful therapeutic option for increasing other targets, such as survival, quality of life, and hospi-talization rate. These data are in line with previous demonstrations by Auricchio and colleagues[9] and suggest that other variables, more strictly related to CO and its increase during exercise, may be more useful than peak VO_2 to assess CRT efficacy.

Few studies suggested that prognostic value of peak VO_2 could be improved by adding other nonin-vasively obtained exercise parameters to peak VO_2 (eg, ventilation efficiency [VE/VCO$_2$ slope])[10–12] and the so-called "peak circulatory power."[11] The latter is considered an index of the work that the heart is able to do while combining CO (which is re-flected by VO_2) and systolic pressure. None of the various proposed combined indexes is a true measurement of CO during exercise because they are only indirectly related to CO.

WHAT CARDIAC OUTPUT MEASUREMENTS ADD TO PROGNOSIS AND THERAPY TAILORING

Griffin and colleagues[13] were the first to show that peak exercise CO-derived parameters were able to predict prognosis in patients who have CHF better than exercise tolerance or peak VO_2. Wilson

Table 1
$C(a-v)O_2$ values at anaerobic threshold

	Class A Peak VO_2 > 20 mL/min/kg	Class B Peak VO_2 15–20 mL/min/kg	Class C Peak VO_2 < 15 mL/min/kg)
$C(a-v)O_2$ at anaerobic threshold mL/100 mL	12.3 ± 1.3*	13.1 ± 2.7	13.4 ± 2.6

* $P < .05$ versus class B and C.
   Data from Agostoni PG, Wasserman K, Perego, et al. Non-invasive measurement of stroke volume during exercise in heart failure patients. Clin Sci (Lond) 2000;98:545–51.

and colleagues,[14] Chomsky and colleagues,[15] and Metra and colleagues[16] confirmed that hemodynamically derived CO parameters at peak exercise have a greater prognostic power than peak VO_2. Metra and colleagues[16] reported that more than 40% of the normal hemodynamic response heart failure subjects had a peak VO_2 of less than 14 mL/min/kg. Consequently, they suggested performing hemodynamic measurements during exercise in heart failure evaluation to avoid heart transplantation for patients whose exercise limitation is caused by muscle deconditioning more than pump failure. The introduction of various useful therapies and the possibility of improving prognosis even in the most compromised patients made it clear that it was not possible to follow a great number of patients with regular invasive hemodynamic evaluation in terms of patient safety, comfort, and use of community resources.

In 2001, Williams and colleagues[17] integrated a standard cardiopulmonary test with noninvasive measurements of CO using CO_2 rebreathing. This method is complicated because the equilibrium between CO_2 in the rebreathing balloon and CO_2 in the blood needs to be reached before the beginning of blood—and inhaled CO_2—recirculation. This process allows only 20 to 30 seconds for the measurement at rest and even less during exercise. CO_2 concentration tanks and balloon dimensions need to be changed according to the stage of the disease and the size of the patients. Ventilation-perfusion mismatch represents a potential technical source of errors. Since then, few studies have been conducted using other noninvasive methods for determination of peak exercise CO, but tests were mainly related to the possibility of measuring CO during exercise in patients who had CHF and not its usefulness for prognosis or therapy tailoring.

Only few data have been published recently regarding the use of CO-derived parameters in the assessment of the therapeutic efficacy of pharmacologic, resynchronization, or surgical therapy. Among those, Schlosshan and colleagues[18] recently evaluated 17 patients who have CHF before and after CRT using measurement of peak VO_2 and peak CO by CO_2 rebreathing technique. Despite the small cohort of patients, the short follow-up (6–8 months), and the methodologic problems, this is the first demonstration of the beneficial hemodynamic effects in terms of the flow- and pressure-generating capacity of the cardiac pump after CRT. Several studies have been conducted regarding surgical or nonsurgical mitral insufficiency repair, but no data on the effects of these procedures on CO during exercise exist. These are only a few examples of the fields that need to be covered by more studies because several questions regarding CO behavior during exercise in patients who have CHF are without answers.

TECHNIQUES AVAILABLE FOR MEASURING CARDIAC OUTPUT DURING EXERCISE

The ideal method for determining CO during a standard exercise test should be safe, reliable, repeatable, and possibly inexpensive. These needs exclude all invasive methods and those that require an invasive approach for calibration purposes, such as pulse CO, which needs a lithium dye dilution technique for calibration.[19] Unfortunately, the noninvasive techniques for CO determination, such as the single-breath acetylene method,[20,21] the carbon dioxide rebreathing methods,[22–25] and methods based on impedance cardiography[26] and pulse contour analysis,[27] have been proven less reliable during exercise. Conversely, inert gas rebreathing (IGR) with continuous analysis of expired gases is a reliable, safe, and inexpensive method for carrying out noninvasive measurements of pulmonary blood flow, which is equivalent to CO in the absence of blood shunts.[28] This method seems promising and may open a new era of CO measurement.

INERT GAS REBREATHING METHOD

Noninvasive CO measure by gas rebreathing is an old method that was introduced by August Krogh in 1912, but it has become a simple and easy-to-use method for measuring CO only with the recent introduction of a small and portable device (Inno-cor Rebreathing System, Innovision A/S, Odense, Denmark). IGR technique uses an oxygen-en-riched mixture of an inert soluble gas (0.5% nitrous oxide) and an inert insoluble gas (0.1% sulfur hex-afluoride) from a prefilled bag (**Fig. 1**). Patients breathe into a respiratory valve via a mouthpiece and a bacterial filter with a nose clip. At the end of expiration, the valve is activated so that patients rebreathe from the prefilled bag for a period of 10 to 20 seconds. After that period, patients are switched back to ambient air and CO measure-ment is terminated. Photo-acoustic analyzers measure gas concentration over a five-breath interval. Sulfur hexafluoride is insoluble in blood and is used to determine the lung volume. Nitrous oxide is soluble in blood, and its concentration decreases during rebreathing with a rate that is proportional to pulmonary blood flow, that is, the blood flow that perfuses the active part of the alveoli.

CO is equal to pulmonary blood flow when the arterial oxygen saturation measure (SpO_2) is high (>98% using the pulse oximeter) showing the absence of pulmonary shunt flow. If SpO_2 is less than 98%, CO is equal to pulmonary blood flow plus shunt flow, which is calculated as follows (**Fig. 2**):

$$Shunt\ flow = CO - PBF \tag{1}$$

$$VO_2 = (CcO_2 - CvO_2) \bullet PBF \tag{2}$$

$$VO_2 = (CaO_2 - CvO_2) \bullet CO \tag{3}$$

Rearranging Equation (2) gives

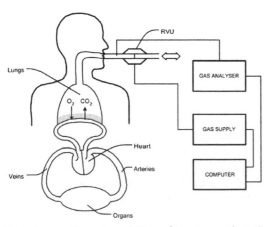

Fig. 1. Schematic representation of inert gas rebreath-ing measurement. RVU, respiratory valve unit. (*Courtesy of* Innovision, Odense, Dennmark; with permission.)

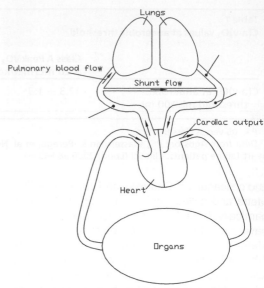

Fig. 2. Schematic representation of shunt flow. (*Courtesy of* Innovision, Odense, Dennmark; with permission.)

$$CvO_2 = CcO_2 - VO_2/PBF$$

Inserting into equation (3) gives

$$CO = VO_2/(CaO_2 - CcO_2 + VO_2/PBF)$$

or

$$CO = 1/[(CaO_2 - CcO_2)/VO_2 + 1/PBF] \tag{4}$$

Insertion Equation (4) in Equation (1) gives us the shunt flow equation

$$1/[(CaO_2 - CcO_2)/VO_2 + 1/PBF] - PBF$$

where CaO_2 equals arterial O_2 content, CvO_2 equals mixed venous O_2 content, and CcO_2 equals end pulmonary capillary O_2 content. VO_2, CO, pulmonary blood flow, CaO_2, and CvO_2 were measured directly, whereas CcO_2 was estimated by assuming that pulmonary capillary O_2 satura-tion equals 98% and using hemoglobin values ob-tained from blood samples.

In two experimental studies, Reinhart and colleagues[29] and Friedman and colleagues[30] showed insensibility of the IGR method to ventila-tion/perfusion mismatch. A clinical study demon-strated the usefulness of the IGR method in patients with pulmonary diseases, evaluating patients with near normal lung function and patients with abnormal lung function able to rebreathe 40% or more of their predicted vital capacity with four or five breaths in 20 seconds.[31]

In 2005, we tested the possibility of measuring CO during exercise by the IGR method in patients who have CHF.[32] After positioning a 7-Fr Swan Ganz catheter in the pulmonary artery and a small catheter in the radial artery, we measured CO at rest and at different steps of exercise of cardiopulmonary exercise testing by IGR, Fick method (F) and thermodilution (T) simultaneously. Repeatability of CO measurement by the IGR method was assessed with a variation coefficient of 10.8%, and a good linear correlation was assessed between CO measurement by F versus T, IGR versus F and IGR versus T (r = 0.96, 0.95, 0.94) and confirmed by Bland and Altman analysis. Our data showed that CO measurement by the IGR method is repeatable and reliable at rest and during exercise in patients who have CHF. Simultaneous measurement of VO_2 and CO during exercise allows calculation of arteriovenous oxygen difference $(C(a-v)O_2)$. In **Fig. 3**, CO is plotted versus $C(a-v)O_2$. The solid lines are $isoVO_2$ lines. Full symbols represent data from the Fick method (measured VO_2, measured $C(a-v)O_2$ and calculated CO), and open symbols represent data from the IGR method (measured CO, measured VO_2, calculated $C(a-v)O_2$), demonstrating the reliability of noninvasive measurements. Plotting these three variables together, it is possible to discriminate exercise limitation caused by altered left ventricle pump function from limitation caused by other factors, including muscle enzyme deficiency and deconditioning.

In 2007, Lang and colleagues[33] assessed the efficacy of the IGR method in 88 patients who had severe CHF. They demonstrated that patients who had CHF were able to rapidly learn the rebreathing technique at rest and during exercise. Eighty-six percent of the test results provided successful measurement of metabolic and CO data, which showed that metabolic stress testing and IGR can be performed easily in patients with CHF.

FUTURE PERSPECTIVES

Currently, we have few data about the clinical use of CO determination during exercise by the IGR technique. We do know that these measurements are feasible, but it is still unclear whether they are useful. We can foresee a use of CO determination during exercise by the IGR technique in several clinical settings, such as determination of the response to cardiac resynchronization, exercise training, or presurgical evaluation of mitral regurgitation. The description of CO behavior during exercise in a large population of normal subjects with different ages and gender is clearly needed.

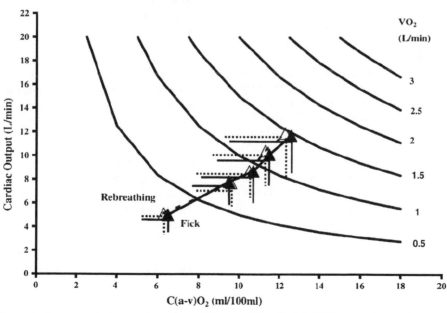

Fig. 3. Cardiac output versus arteriovenous oxygen difference $[C(a-v)O_2]$. Solid lines are $isoVO_2$ lines. Solid symbols represent data obtained from Fick method. Open symbols represent data from the inert gas rebreathing technique. (*From* Agostoni P, Cattadori G, Apostolo A, et al. Noninvasive measurement of cardiac output during exercise by inert gas rebreathing technique: a new tool for heart failure evaluation. J Am Coll Cardiol 2005;46:17780; with permission.)

REFERENCES

1. Stringer WW, Hansen JE, Wasserman K. Cardiac output estimated noninvasively from oxygen uptake during exercise. J Appl Phys 1997;82:908–12.

2. Perego GB, Marenzi GC, Guazzi M, et al. Contribution of PO2, P50, and Hb to changes in arteriovenous O_2 content during exercise in heart failure. J Appl Phys 1996;80:623–31.

3. Agostoni P, Wasserman K, Guazzi M, et al. Exercise-induced hemoconcentration in heart failure due to dilated cardiomyopathy. Am J Cardiol 1999;83:278–80, A276.

4. Agostoni P, Cerino M, Palermo P, et al. Exercise capacity in patients with beta-thalassaemia intermedia. Br J Haematol 2005;131:278–81.

5. Agostoni P, Wasserman K, Perego GB, et al. Oxygen transport to muscle during exercise in chronic congestive heart failure secondary to idiopathic dilated cardiomyopathy. Am J Cardiol 1997;79:1120–4.

6. Agostoni PG, Wasserman K, Perego, et al. Non-invasive measurement of stroke volume during exercise in heart failure patients. Clin Sci (Lond) 2000;98:545–51.

7. Hunt SA. ACC/AHA 2005 guideline update for the diagnosis and management of chronic heart failure in the adult: a report of the American College of Cardiology/American Heart Association task force on practice guidelines (writing committee to update the 2001 guidelines for the evaluation and management of heart failure). J Am Coll Cardiol 2005;46:e1–82.

8. Wasserman K, Sun XG, Hansen JE, et al. Effect of biventricular pacing on the exercise pathophysiology of heart failure. Chest 2007;132:250–61.

9. Auricchio A, Kloss M, Trautmann SI, et al. Exercise performance following cardiac resynchronization therapy in patients with heart failure and ventricular conduction delay. Am J Cardiol 2002;89:198–203.

10. Arena R, Myers J, Aslam SS, et al. Peak VO2 and VE/VCO2 slope in patients with heart failure: a prognostic comparison. Am Heart J 2004;147:354–60.

11. Corra U, Mezzani A, Bosimini E, et al. Cardiopulmonary exercise testing and prognosis in chronic heart failure: a prognosticating algorithm for the individual patient. Chest 2004;126:942–50.

12. Cohen-Solal A, Tabet JY, Logeart D, et al. A non-invasively determined surrogate of cardiac power (circulatory power) at peak exercise is a powerful prognostic factor in chronic heart failure. Eur Heart J 2002;23:806–14.

13. Griffin BP, Shah PK, Ferguson J, et al. Incremental prognostic value of exercise hemodynamic variables in chronic congestive heart failure secondary to coronary artery disease or to dilated cardiomyopathy. Am J Cardiol 1991;67:848–53.

14. Wilson JR, Rayos G, Yeoh TK, et al. Dissociation between peak exercise oxygen consumption and hemodynamic dysfunction in potential heart transplant candidates. J Am Coll Cardiol 1995;26:429–35.

15. Chomsky DB, Lang CC, Rayos GH, et al. Hemodynamic exercise testing: a valuable tool in the selection of cardiac transplantation candidates. Circulation 1996;94:3176–83.

16. Metra M, Faggiano P, D'Aloia A, et al. Use of cardiopulmonary exercise testing with hemodynamic monitoring in the prognostic assessment of ambulatory patients with chronic heart failure. J Am Coll Cardiol 1999;33:943–50.

17. Williams SG, Cooke GA, Wright DJ, et al. Peak exercise cardiac power output: a direct indicator of cardiac function strongly predictive of prognosis in chronic heart failure. Eur Heart J 2001;22:1496–503.

18. Schlossan D, Barker D, Pepper D, et al. CRT improves the exercise capacity and functional reserve of the failing heart through enhancing the cardiac flow- and pressure-generating capacity. Eur J Heart Fail 2006;8(5):515–21.

19. Jonas MM, Tanser SJ. Lithium dilution measurement of cardiac output and arterial pulse waveform analysis: an indicator dilution calibrated beat-by-beat system for continuous estimation of cardiac output. Curr Opin Crit Care 2002;8:257–61.

20. Elkayam U, Wilson AF, Morrison J, et al. Non-invasive measurement of cardiac output by a single breath constant expiratory technique. Thorax 1984;39:107–13.

21. Zenger MR, Brenner M, Haruno M, et al. Measurement of cardiac output by automated single-breath technique, and comparison with thermodilution and Fick methods in patients with cardiac disease. Am J Cardiol 1993;71:105–9.

22. Jones NL, Campbell EJ, McHardy GJ, et al. The estimation of carbon dioxide pressure of mixed venous blood during exercise. Clin Sci 1967;32:311–27.

23. van Herwaarden CL, Binkhorst RA, Fennis JF, et al. Reliability of the cardiac output measurement with the indirect Fick-principle for CO_2 during exercise. Pflugers Arch 1980;385:21–3.

24. Klausen K. Comparison of CO_2 rebreathing and acetylene methods for cardiac output. J Appl Phys 1965;20:763–6.

25. Farhi LE, Nesarajah MS, Olszowka AJ, et al. Cardiac output determination by simple one-step rebreathing technique. Respir Physiol 1976;28:141–59.

26. Sramek BB. Thoracic electrical bioimpedance measurement of cardiac output. Crit Care Med 1994;22:1337–9.

27. Stok WJ, Baisch F, Hillebrecht A, et al. Noninvasive cardiac output measurement by arterial pulse analysis compared with inert gas rebreathing. J Appl Phys 1993;74:2687–93.

28. Sackner MA, Greeneltch D, Heiman MS, et al. Diffusing capacity, membrane diffusing capacity, capillary blood volume, pulmonary tissue volume, and cardiac output measured by a rebreathing technique. Am Rev Respir Dis 1975;111:157–65.

29. Reinhart ME, Hughes JR, Kung M, et al. Determination of pulmonary blood flow by the rebreathing technique in airflow obstruction. Am Rev Respir Dis 1979;120:533–40.

30. Friedman M, Wilkins SA Jr, Rothfeld AF, et al. Effect of ventilation and perfusion imbalance on inert gas rebreathing variables. J Appl Phys 1984;56:364–9.

31. Kallay MC, Hyde RW, Smith RJ, et al. Cardiac output by rebreathing in patients with cardiopulmonary diseases. J Appl Phys 1987;63:201–10.

32. Agostoni P, Cattadori G, Apostolo A, et al. Noninvasive measurement of cardiac output during exercise by inert gas rebreathing technique: a new tool for heart failure evaluation. J Am Coll Cardiol 2005;46:1779–81.

33. Lang CC, Karlin P, Haythe J, et al. Ease of noninvasive measurement of cardiac output coupled with peak VO_2 determination at rest and during exercise in patients with heart failure. Am J Cardiol 2007;99: 404–5.

Invasive Hemodynamic Assessment in Heart Failure

Barry A. Borlaug, MD[a],*, David A. Kass, MD[b]

KEYWORDS

- Hemodynamics • Heart failure • Systole • Diastole
- Ventricular-arterial interaction • Cardiovascular function

The concept of hemodynamics was born in 1628 with Harvey's description of the circulation, but its growth was limited for centuries by the inability to measure pressure and flow accurately. The work of Starling, Wiggers, and other hemodynamic physiologists in the first part of the twentieth century, along with introduction of cardiac catheterization by Cournand and Richards in the 1940s ushered in the golden era of hemodynamics. From the late 1970s to early 1990s, there was an explosion of clinical and basic research as new methods were developed to quantify ventricular systolic and diastolic properties more definitively. Enthusiasm for such characterization subsequently waned, however, as therapies directly targeting hemodynamic derangements, such as inotropes, were found to hasten mortality. This change coincided with a paradigm shift in the way heart failure was conceptualized, from a disease of abnormal hemodynamics to one of neurohormonal derangements, abnormal cell signaling, and maladaptive remodeling. As such, many "gold-standard" methods for characterizing load, contractility, diastole, and, ventricular-arterial interaction were not adopted into clinical practice. A working understanding of each element remains paramount to interpret properly the hemodynamic changes in patients who have acute and chronic heart failure, however.

Routine cardiac catheterization provides data on left heart, right heart, systemic and pulmonary arterial pressures, vascular resistances, cardiac output, and ejection fraction. These data are often then applied as markers of cardiac preload, afterload, and global function, although each of these parameters reflects more complex interactions between the heart and its internal and external loads. This article reviews more specific, gold standard assessments of ventricular and arterial properties and how these relate to the parameters reported and used in practice, and then discusses the re-emerging importance of invasive hemodynamics in the assessment and management of heart failure.

CARDIAC CONTRACTILITY: LOOKING BEYOND THE EJECTION FRACTION

The most universally accepted index of contractility used in practice, the EF, unfortunately is also one of the least specific.[1] As with any parameter measuring the extent of muscle shortening or thickening, it is highly sensitive to afterload and really is an expression of ventricular-arterial coupling rather than of contractility alone. EF also is affected by heart size, because its denominator is end-diastolic volume (EDV), leading many to propose that EF is more a parameter of remodeling than of contractility. EF commonly is used to classify different "forms" of heart failure (low versus preserved EF).[2] This approach is appealing, given its binary nature and ease of application in practice, but the realities of how a patient develops signs and symptoms of heart failure are far more complex,[3] and in this regard EF serves as a somewhat arbitrary marker.

More specific measures of contractility have been developed but because of their complexity

[a] Mayo Clinic and Foundation, Rochester, MN, USA
[b] Johns Hopkins Medical Institutions, Baltimore, MD, USA
* Corresponding author. Division of Cardiovascular Diseases, Department of Medicine, Mayo Clinic and Foundation, Gonda 5-455, 200 First Street SW, Rochester, MN 55905.
E-mail address: borlaug.barry@mayo.edu (B.A. Borlaug).

Heart Failure Clin 5 (2009) 217–228
doi:10.1016/j.hfc.2008.11.008
1551-7136/08/$ – see front matter © 2009 Elsevier Inc. All rights reserved

remain used principally in research. The maximal rate of pressure rise during isovolumic contraction (dP/dt$_{max}$) can be assessed using a high-fidelity micromanometer and is used widely as a measure of contractility. dP/dt$_{max}$, however, is dependent on cardiac filling (ie, is preload dependent) and heart rate, and it may not always reflect contractile function that develops after cardiac ejection is initiated.[4] In patients who have cardiac dyssynchrony, the lack of coordinated contraction in early-systole reduces dP/dt$_{max}$ because the force developed by the early activated wall is dissipated by stretching of the still relaxed opposite wall.[5] dP/dt$_{max}$ is quite sensitive to this phenomenon (**Fig. 1**), but in this case it reflects chamber mechanics rather than intrinsic muscle function.

An ideal parameter of contractility would assess inotropic state independently of preload, afterload, heart rate, and remodeling.[1] This assessment still

remains somewhat elusive, but parameters derived from relations between cardiac pressure and volume have come the closest to achieving it. As shown in **Fig. 1B**, a series of variably loaded pressure–volume (PV) loops can be obtained to assess systolic, diastolic, coupling, and energetic properties. Stroke work, dP/dt$_{max}$, maximal ventricular power, elastance, efficiency, and other parameters are assessed, and by examining these variables over a range of preload volumes, one can derive more load-independent, cardiac-specific measures.[6]

The relationship between end-systolic pressure and volume from a variety of variably loaded cardiac contractions yields the end-systolic pressure–volume relationship (ESPVR),[7] its slope being the end-systolic elastance (Ees) (see **Fig. 1B**). The Ees conveys information about both contractile function and myocardial

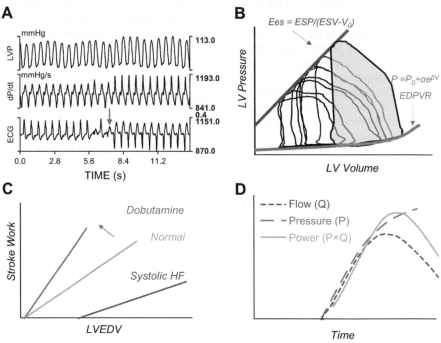

Fig. 1. (*A*) Time plot of left ventricular pressure (LVP), first derivative of pressure (dP/dt), and EKG in a patient who has heart failure with left bundle-type conduction delay. At the arrow, the patient received bi-ventricular stimulation resulting in an abrupt rise in dP/dt$_{max}$. (*B*) PV loops obtained at baseline and during transient caval occlusion (decreasing LV volumes—loops moving right to left). The slope of the EDSPV derived from multibeat analysis defines ventricular Ees, a load-independent measure of contractility. By measuring diastolic pressure and volume during diastasis at variably loaded beats, the end-diastolic PV relationship (EDPVR) is obtained. The shaded area subtended by the baseline loop represents the stroke work performed by the ventricle. ESP, end-systolic pressure; ESV, end-systolic volume; V$_0$, volume axis intercept of ESPVR. (*C*) The slope of the relation between systolic chamber performance (stroke work) and preload (left ventricle end-diastolic volume, LVEDV) determines the preload recruitable stroke work. This relationship shifts up and to the left, as indicated by the arrow, with an increase in contractility, as with dobutamine, or down and to the right with systolic heart failure (HF). (*D*) LV power (P × Q, *solid line*) is determined by the product of simultaneously measured pressure (P, *dashed line*) and flow (Q, *dotted line*). When indexed to preload, this calculation produces another load-independent measure of LV chamber contractility.

constitutive properties; that is, it is a measure of chamber stiffness. It can be related easily to arterial vascular load to assess ventricular–arterial interaction[8] and provides important information about how a patient's blood pressure and flow will respond to loading changes.[9] Although traditionally Ees was assessed from multiple cardiac cycles requiring simultaneous measurement of cardiac pressure and volume (or flow), algorithms have been generated and tested to derive these parameters noninvasively from single steady-state data.[10–12] These parameters have been used to characterize systolic properties in various forms of heart failure and in larger populations.[6,13,14] The diastolic correlate of Ees is the end-diastolic elastance, the lower PV boundary that is parameterized most often by a mono-exponential stiffness coefficient. Both the Ees and diastolic curve fits are dependent on chamber size and remodeling.

Several other parameters commonly are derived for indexing systolic function. The relationship between stroke work and preload, measured from multiple beats under different loading generates a "Sarnoff curve," and its slope, often termed "preload recruitable stroke work" (PRSW) provides a contractile index (see **Fig. 1**C).[15] Maximal ventricular power (PWR$_{max}$) is the peak instantaneous product of ventricular outflow and pressure and also is quite preload dependent (see **Fig. 1**D).

Regression over a range of preloads yields a more specific index, however, and because the intercept of this relation often is near zero for normal-sized ventricles, the ratio of PWR$_{max}$/EDV can be used. In failing ventricles, normalization to EDV^2 seems to reduce load dependence better.[16,17]

DIASTOLE—MORE THAN END-DIASTOLIC PRESSURE

Diastolic function is determined from active and passive processes, and both contribute to relaxation and chamber filling.[3] Left heart filling pressures, either pulmonary artery occlusion (wedge pressure) or left ventricle (LV) end-diastolic pressure (EDP), are central to standard cardiac catheterization, and their elevation is taken to reflect abnormal loading and/or abnormal chamber compliance. One cannot determine whether the elevation reflects abnormal loading or abnormal chamber compliance from the pressure parameter alone, but diastolic function also is assessed by a variety of noninvasive methods to characterize it better.

Aortic valve closure marks the onset of ventricular diastole, where relaxation is quantified invasively by the rate of pressure decay, typically expressed by a time constant (τ) that is estimated using a number of mathematical fits (**Fig. 2**).[18]

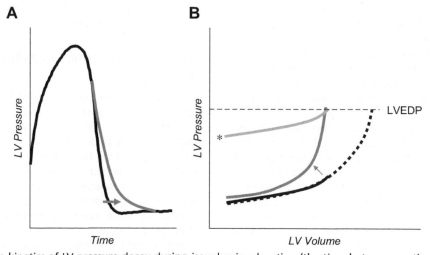

Fig. 2. (*A*) The kinetics of LV pressure decay during isovolumic relaxation (the time between aortic valve closure and mitral opening) can be modeled by various equations to derive the time constant, τ. The curve indicated by the arrow shows prolonged relaxation, often seen with heart failure, aging, and hypertension. (*B*) Groups of DPVR. The solid black line shows the curve in a normal person. The curve that shifts up and to the left (*arrow*) indicates the effects of increased passive chamber stiffness. Filling pressures (LVEDP) may be elevated because of the increased passive chamber stiffness, but similar elevations also can be seen in the absence of increased stiffness, as when there is with increased extrinsic restraint (line indicated by the asterisk). Note that the shape (stiffness) of the DPVR with enhanced restraint is similar to that in the normal patient. Finally, EDP may be elevated simply because of the overfilling of a structurally normal ventricle (*dotted black line*). There is evidence to support each of these possible contributors to elevated EDP in HFpEF.

Even this seemingly straightforward assessment has technical pitfalls. These model fits—usually mono-exponential decays (ie, $P = P_\infty + P_o e^{-t/\tau}$, or the same equation without P_∞)—may or may not describe adequately the actual fall of pressure. When used in a setting where they do not fit properly, such as in dilated heart failure, they can lead to erroneous conclusions.[18] An alternative model based on a modified logistic equation, $P = P_A/(1 + e^{t/\tau}) + P_B$,[19] fits such failure data better than the exponential. Chung and Kovacs[20] recently explored both model fits in contrast to a more physics-based approach, showing that relaxation is best described using both resistive and elastic elements. This intriguing approach deserves further attention in clinical studies.

Delayed relaxation is common. It frequently accompanies normal aging,[21] but it becomes even more prominent in cardiac failure and with hypertrophy. It has multiple determinants starting with dissociation of the cross-bridge, calcium-handling, and elasticity-restoring forces resulting from the recoil of compressed macromolecules such as titin.[3] The extent to which delayed relaxation alters mean and late-diastolic pressures remains controversial,[22] because diastole generally is long enough that even delayed relaxation is completed before late-diastolic filling occurs. It clearly can affect early filling and pressures, particularly at faster heart rates. Analysis requires invasive high-fidelity micromanometer recordings, although it may be approximated by the time between aortic valve closure and mitral valve opening or inferred from mitral Doppler flow patterns.[23]

Similar to isovolumic relaxation, passive diastolic chamber stiffness rarely is measured directly in standard clinical practice. As noted, the LV diastolic pressure–volume relationship (DPVR; see Fig. 1B) is curvilinear; thus compliance most often is expressed by a mono-exponential stiffness coefficient.[24] Linear approximations have been used, but one must be careful to compare these approximations within similar loading ranges. The DPVR most often is estimated from a single heartbeat, although this estimation combines features that reflect early relaxation and resistive (viscous) properties and extra-chamber (eg, pericardial) loading. A more accurate approach is to assess multiple PV loops over a loading range (varying preload) and to connect points at late-diastole from these cycles (see Fig. 1B). The apparent chamber stiffness derived from single versus multiple loops can vary substantially, as shown particularly in patients who have genetic hypertrophic cardiomyopathy; in these patients the use of a single loop markedly underestimated LV stiffness.[25]

LVEDP may be increased because chamber is stiffer or is subject to higher preload or because the entire DPVR is shifted upwards (see Fig. 2B).[3] All three variables play a role in heart failure with a reduced EF. The first and last seem to contribute mostly to heart failure with a preserved EF (HFpEF),[14,26,27] and although some have found increased LV filling volumes as well,[28] this phenomenon has not been seen by others.[14,29] Approximately 40% of a measured intracavitary LV pressure stems from extrinsic forces applied to the LV, mediated by the pericardium and right heart across the interventricular septum.[30] This phenomenon of diastolic ventricular interaction becomes more important as heart size increases (ie, as pericardial space decreases).[31] Even though the LV chamber size usually is normal in HFpEF, total epicardial heart size can be enlarged substantially because of increased atrial size and cardiac hypertrophy, so the pericardial constraint can be relevant.[29] This effect is supported by invasive data from patients who have HFpEF in which the DPVR shifted upwards in patients subjected to exertional stress.[32] In heart failure with low EF, cardiac enlargement in almost all chambers exacerbates pericardial constraint.[31,33] Overfilling of right-sided chambers can increase left-sided pressures via right ventricular (RV)–LV crosstalk as the distending (transmural) pressure that drives LV filling becomes impaired.[34] This mechanism can explain how acute unloading of the right heart paradoxically can increase LV filling and output in patients who have advanced systolic heart failure or cor pulmonale.[33]

AFTERLOAD AND VENTRICULAR–ARTERIAL INTERACTION

Adequate pressure and flow to the body depends both on cardiac performance and on the nature of the vascular load into which it ejects. This load traditionally has been conceived of as equivalent to mean or systolic blood pressure, although this notion can lead to ambiguous interpretations. Unlike isolated muscle (for which the term "afterload" was first defined), where one can fix a constant force during contraction, the intact heart generates varying stress (and pressures) during ejection, and the blood pressure generated is determined as much by the heart's properties as by those of the vasculature.[35] A useful alternative parameter is aortic input impedance, which characterizes the mean and pulsatile properties of the vascular loading circuit and is independent of the heart. Impedance is derived from Fourier analysis of aortic pressure and flow waves,[36,37] traditionally assessed by invasive catheters although noninvasive methods also have been described.

Coupling of impedance to a heart property is mathematically complicated, because impedance is described in the frequency domain (ie, Fourier spectra), and the heart property is described in the time domain. In the early 1980s, however, Sunagawa and colleagues[38,39] developed the parameter effective arterial elastance (Ea), based on LV pressure–volume loop analysis. Ea, like Ees, is measured in units of elastance and can be calculated more easily to study ventricular–arterial interaction. Ea is not a measure of a specific vascular property per se but combines both mean and pulsatile loading (and heart rate influences), providing a lumped parameter reflecting the net impact of this load on the heart. Kelly and colleagues[40] showed that the simple ratio of end-systolic pressure to stroke volume accurately estimates Ea in both hypertensive and normal humans. Graphically Ea is identified by the negative slope running through the end-systolic PV coordinates and EDV at zero pressure (**Fig. 3**). As discussed earlier, LV Ees is determined by the slope of the ESPVR. The Ees reflects chamber

contractility but also is influenced by chamber size and remodeling. Knowledge of Fes, Ea, and EDV allows one to predict blood pressure, stroke volume and stroke work, and EF.[8]

Ees and Ea are matched in healthy persons to provide optimal mechanical efficiency in the transfer of blood from the heart to the body, so that the coupling ratio (Ea/Ees) approaches unity.[41] It can be shown mathematically that the EF varies inversely with the Ea/Ees ratio.[8] In systolic heart failure, contractility (Ees) is low, whereas afterload (Ea) usually is high in the setting of vasoconstriction and neurohormonal activation. This condition produces "afterload mismatch" so that the coupling ratio increases, meaning that the EF decreases.[42] With advanced systolic dysfunction, it usually is difficult to increase contractility (Ees) effectively because of limited inotropic reserve, but therapies reducing Ea to very low levels have been extremely useful in optimizing ventricular ejection in such patients.

Conceptualizing systolic heart failure in terms of ventricular–arterial interaction can help explain the

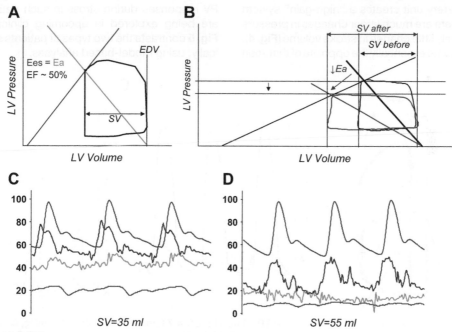

Fig. 3. (A) Normal steady-state PV loop. Ea is defined by the negative slope (*green line*) running between the end-systolic PV point and EDV at *P* = 0. In healthy persons, Ees (*red line*) and Ea are matched to maintain optimal coupling and efficiency, with an EF of around 50% to 60% when the volume intercept is near zero. (B) In systolic heart failure, the heart is dilated (increased EDV), Ees is low (shallow ESPVR), and the EF is reduced. Acute reduction of Ea with a vasodilator (*red*) leads to a marked 50% increase in stroke volume (SV after) with very little reduction in blood pressure. (C) Radial artery (*red*), pulmonary artery (*blue*), pulmonary wedge (*green*), and right atrial (*pink*) pressure versus time in a patient who has dilated cardiomyopathy. There is severe pulmonary arterial and venous hypertension with borderline systemic hypotension. SV, stroke volume. (D) The same patient on a high dose (7 μg/kg/min) of sodium nitroprusside. Note the near-normalization of cardiac filling pressures with marked increase in stroke volume (SV), with little change in systolic blood pressure.

clinical response to vasodilator therapy of patients who have dilated cardiomyopathy.[9] **Fig. 3**B shows a typical resting PV loop from such a patient. Because of the shallow slope of the ESPVR (low Ees), there is little change in blood pressure despite a marked improvement in stroke volume for a given dose of vasodilator. **Fig. 3**C and D shows pressure tracings as part of transplant evaluation for a patient who has advanced dilated cardiomyopathy. Filling pressures are high at baseline, pulmonary vascular resistance is prohibitively elevated, and there is systemic hypotension. With the administration of sodium nitroprusside there is marked improvement in cardiac output, filling pressures, and pulmonary vascular resistance and no significant reduction in systolic pressures—all as predicted based on the principals of ventricular–arterial coupling.

Although the coupling ratio is useful for determining stroke volume and the pressure generated during systole, the absolute magnitude of both the numerator and denominator is equally important. In normal aging, systolic hypertension, and renal disease, there are exaggerated increases in both ventricular and vascular stiffness.[8] The stiff ventricle-artery unit creates a "high-gain" system in which there are much larger changes in pressure with relatively little change in stroke volume (**Fig. 4**). This situation is essentially the opposite of that seen in systolic heart failure, where loading changes result in relatively minor alterations in blood pressure, despite more dramatic changes in stroke volume. The importance in ventricular-arterial stiffening becomes most dramatic in many patients who have HFpEF, who can have quite high Ea and Ees.[32] **Fig. 4**B and C shows LV and pulmonary artery pressures from a typical patient who has HFpEF and increased ventricular-arterial stiffness. At rest (see **Fig. 4**B), there is severe systemic and pulmonary artery hypertension. In contrast to the patient who has heart failure and low EF shown in **Fig. 3**, there is a marked hypotensive effect after the administration of a very low dose of nitroprusside (see **Fig. 4**C) with little or no change in stroke volume and cardiac output. In this way, high resting stiffness greatly amplified the change in blood pressure for a given change in preload or afterload while minimizing changes in stroke volume. Increased ventricular-arterial stiffening helps explain the clinical behavior of patients who have HFpEF, who often oscillate between hypertensive crisis and symptomatic hypotension with relatively minor perturbations. Treatments targeting combined stiffening may allow better regulation of PV responses during stress in such patients and are being explored in upcoming clinical trials.[3] **Fig. 5** contrasts the two types of patients schematically, using model-based analyses.

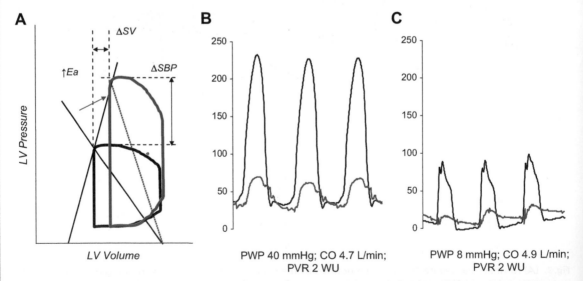

A

↑Ea   ΔSV   ΔSBP

LV Pressure

LV Volume

B

PWP 40 mmHg; CO 4.7 L/min; PVR 2 WU

C

PWP 8 mmHg; CO 4.9 L/min; PVR 2 WU

Fig. 4. (*A*) With aging, hypertension, and in HFpEF, ventricular (Ees) and arterial (Ea) stiffness increases. Although the Ea/Ees ratio may remain normal, combined ventricular and vascular stiffening leads to marked fluctuations in blood pressure with relatively small changes in preload or afterload. This condition is in striking contrast to heart failure with low EF (see **Fig. 3**B). (*B*) LV (*black*) and pulmonary artery (*red*) pressure tracings from an 81-year-old woman who has HFpEF demonstrating severe systemic and pulmonary artery hypertension, with markedly elevated LVEDP and wedge pressures (not shown). (*C*) In response to a very low dose of sodium nitroprusside (2 μg), filling pressures normalize, but severe hypotension develops. Note that there is little change in cardiac output (stroke volume) with vasodilation, again in striking contrast to heart failure with reduced EF. CO, cardiac output; PVR, pulmonary vascular resistance; PWP, pulmonary wedge pressure; WU, Wood units.

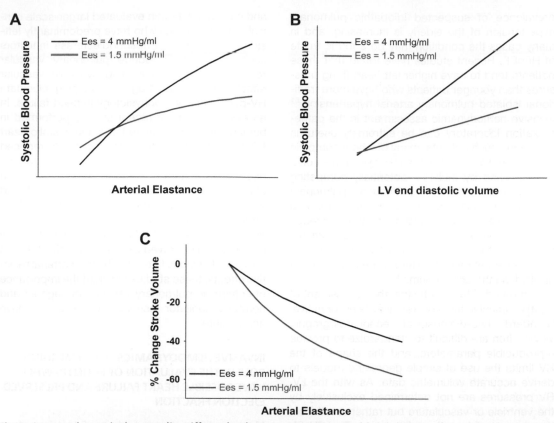

Fig. 5. Increased ventricular systolic stiffness leads to a greater rise in blood pressure for a given increase in (A) afterload or (B) preload. (C) Although isolated increases in afterload lead to a predictable reduction in stroke volume for a given level of contractility, this afterload dependence is more marked in patients who have lower Ees, as seen in patients who have heart failure with reduced EF.

Arterial–ventricular interaction also is important in affecting diastolic processes. Acutely increased vascular load, particularly applied in late ventricular systole,[43] prolongs relaxation in humans and animals.[3,44] Such load dependence becomes more pronounced in heart failure, perhaps related in part to abnormal phosphorylation of sarcomeric proteins. Troponin I phosphorylation by protein kinase A attenuates afterload-induced impairment in early-diastolic relaxation, and mice lacking such phosphorylation sites have enhanced load-dependent relaxation delay.[45] Acute increases in Ea also have been shown to increase LV diastolic stiffness in an aged canine model of HFpEF.[46] LV early-diastolic relaxation varies inversely with net afterload and vascular stiffness in humans with and without hypertensive heart disease[43] and is correlated most closely with pulsatile components, particularly late-systolic load, determined by returning pressure wave reflections and arterial stiffening.

THE RIGHT HEART

Pulmonary hypertension and accompanying right heart dysfunction is increasingly common in patients who have heart failure, regardless of EF, and potently affect exercise capacity and clinical outcome.[47,48] Pulmonary hypertension generally is defined as a mean pulmonary arterial pressure higher than 25 mm Hg at rest (30 mm Hg with exercise), whereas pulmonary arterial hypertension (ie, pulmonary vascular disease) further requires an elevated pulmonary vascular resistance while maintaining a normal pulmonary capillary wedge pressure.[49] The presence of pulmonary vascular resistance and the ability to reduce it with vasodilators are used commonly to establish eligibility for cardiac transplantation. Drug testing uses nitric oxide donators or milrinone and, more recently, the phosphodiesterase 5 inhibitor sildenafil and the natriuretic peptide nesiritide.[50] Although pulmonary artery pressures can be estimated by echo-Doppler methods, invasive assessment is required for definitive diagnosis and to guide treatment decisions.[49]

With the wide use of echo-Doppler cardiography, pulmonary hypertension now is being recognized increasingly, particularly among the older patients presenting with dypsnea.[51] The prevalence of suspected idiopathic pulmonary hypertension of the elderly is increasing, and in many cases the condition may be a forme fruste of HFpEF. Recent studies have found that these patients tend to have higher left heart filling pressures than younger patients who have more traditional isolated pulmonary arterial hypertension.[51] Invasive hemodynamic assessment in the catheterization laboratory can be extremely useful in evaluating such patients, many of whom complain of exertional dyspnea and whose symptoms could be explained by multiple, potentially competing causes (eg, diastolic dysfunction, pulmonary vascular disease, obesity, deconditioning, and others). Interpreting elevated pulmonary wedge pressures in such patients often is difficult, because in the setting of right heart and left atrial enlargement enhanced extrinsic pressure may be applied via the pericardium.[31]

Compared with the left side, the assessment of right ventricular function remains fairly primitive. Standard two-dimensional echocardiographic views often are difficult to standardize to provide reproducible parameters, and the shape of the RV limits the use of simple geometric models to derive accurate volumetric data. As with the LV, RV pressures are not determined exclusively by the ventricle or vasculature but rather result from the dynamic interaction of the two. The RV PV loop normally is triangular, reflecting the lower resistive load and relatively higher compliance of the pulmonary vascular circuit, although it becomes more rectangular (like the LV) in patients who have pulmonary hypertension (perhaps making application of standard LV approaches and the assumptions behind them more justified in this setting). Assessment of RV diastolic stiffness is quite rare in the literature and is affected greatly by pericardial restraint and biventricular remodeling. RV vascular impedance consists of mean pulmonary resistance, the proximal stiffness of pulmonary conduit arteries, characteristic impedance, distal vascular compliance, and reflected waves. There now is renewed interest in how these properties of impedance can impose late-systolic loads on the RV[52] (much as they do on the LV), impacting RV remodeling, relaxation delay, and inefficiency.

The importance of the right heart–pulmonary vascular interaction on symptoms in chronic heart failure is appreciated increasingly. Traditional vasodilators used to treat heart failure (eg, converting enzyme inhibitors and angiotensin receptor blockers) tend to have less effect on the pulmonary circuit. Treatments used to target the pulmonary vasculature, such as prostacyclin and endothelin antagonists, also have systemic effects and have not yet been evaluated larger-scale clinical trials in patients who have predominantly left-sided heart failure. Phosphodiesterase inhibitors such as sildenafil reduce pulmonary vascular resistance while having mild systemic vascular effects, and these drugs are helping elucidate RV-pulmonary pathophysiology in heart failure. In an elegant series of recent studies performed in humans who had primary left-sided systolic heart failure, sildenafil acutely and chronically reduced pulmonary resistance, correlating with enhanced exercise capacity, without much systemic change.[53,54] In another study, investigators found sildenafil improved endothelial function (flow-mediated dilation) in addition to reducing pulmonary resistance, and this improvement also was coupled with improved exercise capacity.[55] Given the lack of obvious left-sided heart or arterial resistive effects, these studies highlight the importance of enhancing pulmonary vascular throughput and normal vasodilator reserve in patients who have heart failure.

INVASIVE HEMODYNAMICS: A RE-EMERGING ROLE IN THE EVALUATION OF PATIENTS WHO HAVE POSSIBLE HEART FAILURE AND PRESERVED EJECTION FRACTION

Most cardiologists are fairly confident in making the diagnosis of heart failure when a patient who has severe LV enlargement and an EF of 25% presents with dyspnea, but a significant group of patients present with exertional dyspnea, clinical euvolemia (or only mild hypervolemia), and a normal EF. The differential diagnosis is fairly broad, including noncardiac causes (deconditioning, obesity, anemia, and other possibilities) and a variety of cardiogenic sources. These conditions may include valvular disease, isolated right heart failure, pulmonary vascular disease, constrictive pericarditis, restrictive cardiomyopathy, or "garden variety" HFpEF. The correct diagnosis often can be made from the combination of physical examination, comprehensive echo-Doppler evaluation, and plasma natriuretic peptide levels. In many patients, particularly the elderly, the picture is not so clear, because diastolic dysfunction seen on echo-Doppler imaging is common in this cohort,[21] and natriuretic peptide levels may be mildly elevated even in the absence of true heart failure.[56]

Invasive hemodynamic assessment in the catheterization laboratory can be clinically useful in these cases. Fig. 6 shows hemodynamics from an 80-year-old woman who has class II-III dyspnea, normal EF, mild diastolic dysfunction, and mild to moderate pulmonary hypertension on

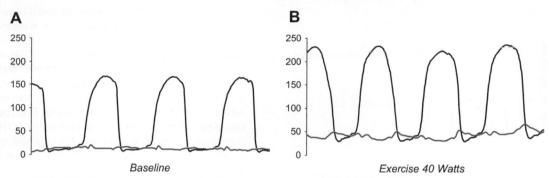

Fig. 6. (A) LV (*black*) and pulmonary wedge (*red*) pressures at rest in a patient who has symptoms of New York Heart Association class II-III dyspnea and normal LV size and function on echocardiogram. Despite mild to moderate systemic hypertension, cardiac filling pressures are normal, arguing against heart failure. (B) With low-level (40 W) supine exercise in the catheterization laboratory, there is a dramatic increase in cardiac filling pressures (to 45–50 mm Hg) associated with significant dyspnea, suggesting that HFpEF indeed is the cause of the patient's symptoms.

echocardiogram. Filling pressures are normal at rest (see **Fig. 6**A), suggesting that the patient's symptoms may not be related to heart failure. Supine exercise at low workload (see **Fig. 6**B), however, reveals a marked increase in cardiac filling pressures associated with severe symptoms of dyspnea. Pulmonary artery pressures increase in proportion to the increase in pulmonary wedge, indicating that the patient's symptoms probably are caused primarily by HFpEF. Other patients may show filling pressures and cardiac output that are normal both at rest and at maximal workload, arguing against a diagnosis of HFpEF. Finally, others develop pulmonary arterial hypertension with exercise in the absence of an increase in left heart filling pressures, identifying a more isolated lesion at the level of the pulmonary vasculature. In practice, individual patients may embody any of these conditions or, more commonly, present with some combination of all three, and future research is required to understand how best to treat patients who have each type of response.

Patients who have had cardiac surgery or radiation therapy may present months to years later with predominant right-sided heart failure, and high-fidelity cardiac catheterization focusing on relationships between intrathoracic–intracardiac pressure dissociation and diastolic ventricular interaction can identify whether symptoms are caused predominantly by constrictive physiology, valvular disease, or restrictive cardiomyopathy.[57,58] Administration of arterial vasodilators such as nitroprusside can be useful to determine whether elevated filling pressures are caused by a partially load-dependent process, such as diastolic dysfunction, or an irreversible myopathic process, such as restrictive cardiomyopathy.

Right heart catheterization can be useful in the management of patients who have acute decompensated heart failure, particularly in the setting of right-sided congestion, low cardiac output, and worsening renal function, when central hemodynamic status remains uncertain. In addition, central hemodynamics may provide independent prognostic value in patients who have heart failure. Each of these topics is discussed elsewhere in this issue.

The time course of ventricular stiffening (ie, elastance varying over time, long a bio-engineering concept[59] but with little apparent interest to physicians) could become clinically important in the near future. Novel therapies targeting myofilament calcium sensitivity and/or the filaments (activators) themselves to increase force generation without altering activator calcium or stimulating cAMP/protein kinase A (PKA) cascades are in development.[60] Although phosphorylation of myosin-binding protein C augments early dP/dt_{max} downstream of β-adrenergic stimulation,[4] sensitizers/activators do not work in this manner. Instead of affecting isovolumic contraction, these drugs often enhance myocardial stiffening (elastance), prolonging the time for elastance to reach its peak and thus making the ejection time longer. The difference in mechanisms is not easily discerned from traditional methods of analysis but is shown readily by the elastance curves. **Fig. 7** shows a schematic of such curves comparing the effects of a beta-agonist to a Ca^{2+}-sensitizer. The beta-agonist increases the rate of rise and fall of myocardial stiffening but shortens systole. In contrast, the sensitizer has little effect on the rates of rise and fall but prolongs ejection. The lure of sensitizers is their potential to provide inotropy without the increases in heart rate, risk of

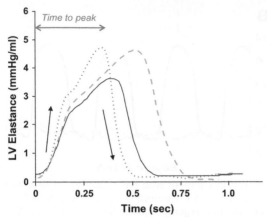

Fig. 7. Time varying elastance curves obtained at baseline (*solid line*), after β-adrenergic stimulation (*dotted line*), and in response to an agent that enhances myofilament calcium sensitivity (*dashed line*). Although the calcium sensitizer has less effect on the early rise in elastance, there is an increase in the time to peak elastance and systolic duration. See text for details.

arrhythmia, or metabolic demand seen with traditional cAMP/PKA-mediated agonists. Such drugs are being developed, so this type of hemodynamic analysis, or a simplified version of it, ultimately may provide ways to index and follow the effects of these drugs in individual patients.

SUMMARY

A few years after fading from the forefront of cardiology, interest in cardiovascular hemodynamics is returning, especially as newer devices are developed that help measure these parameters in patients chronically. Invasive assessment of cardiovascular properties provides greater insight into the mechanisms of disease in disorders such as HFpEF and can explain how patients who have different forms of heart failure respond to various therapies or to certain forms of stress. This information may be useful for treating individual patients and in understanding group differences and treatment effects. Invasive hemodynamic assessment remains the reference standard for assessing systolic and diastolic function and ventricular–arterial interaction and can allow more definitive diagnosis of heart failure, especially in patients where the diagnosis of HF that is based upon clinical and oninvasive evaluation alone remains uncertain.

REFERENCES

1. Kass DA, Maughan WL, Guo ZM, et al. Comparative influence of load versus inotropic states on indexes of ventricular contractility: experimental and theoretical analysis based on pressure-volume relationships. Circulation 1987;76(6):1422–36.

2. Hunt SA, Abraham WT, Chin MH, et al. ACC/AHA 2005 guideline update for the diagnosis and management of chronic heart failure in the adult: a report of the American College of Cardiology/ American Heart Association Task Force on Practice Guidelines (Writing Committee to Update the 2001 Guidelines for the Evaluation and Management of Heart Failure): developed in collaboration with the American College of Chest Physicians and the International Society for Heart and Lung Transplantation: endorsed by the Heart Rhythm Society. Circulation 2005;112(12):e154–235.

3. Borlaug BA, Kass DA. Mechanisms of diastolic dysfunction in heart failure. Trends Cardiovasc Med 2006;16(8):273–9.

4. Nagayama T, Takimoto E, Sadayappan S, et al. Control of in vivo left ventricular [correction] contraction/relaxation kinetics by myosin binding protein C: protein kinase A phosphorylation dependent and independent regulation. Circulation 2007;116(21): 2399–408.

5. Spragg DD, Kass DA. Pathobiology of left ventricular dyssynchrony and resynchronization. Prog Cardiovasc Dis 2006;49(1):26–41.

6. Baicu CF, Zile MR, Aurigemma GP, et al. Left ventricular systolic performance, function, and contractility in patients with diastolic heart failure. Circulation 2005;111(18):2306–12.

7. Suga H, Sagawa K. Instantaneous pressure-volume relationships and their ratio in the excised, supported canine left ventricle. Circ Res 1974;35(1): 117–26.

8. Borlaug BA, Kass DA. Ventricular-vascular interaction in heart failure. Heart Fail Clin 2008;4(1):23–36.

9. Kass DA, Maughan WL. From 'Emax' to pressure-volume relations: a broader view. Circulation 1988; 77(6):1203–12.

10. Chen CH, Fetics B, Nevo E, et al. Noninvasive single-beat determination of left ventricular end-systolic elastance in humans. J Am Coll Cardiol 2001;38(7):2028–34.

11. Lee WS, Huang WP, Yu WC, et al. Estimation of preload recruitable stroke work relationship by a single-beat technique in humans. Am J Physiol Heart Circ Physiol 2003;284(2):H744–50.

12. Borlaug BA, Melenovsky V, Marhin T, et al. Sildenafil inhibits beta-adrenergic-stimulated cardiac contractility in humans. Circulation 2005;112(17):2642–9.

13. Redfield MM, Jacobsen SJ, Borlaug BA, et al. Age- and gender-related ventricular-vascular stiffening: a community-based study. Circulation 2005; 112(15):2254–62.

14. Lam CS, Roger VL, Rodeheffer RJ, et al. Cardiac structure and ventricular-vascular function in

persons with heart failure and preserved ejection fraction from olmsted county, Minnesota. Circulation 2007;115(15):1982–90.

15. Glower DD, Spratt JA, Snow ND, et al. Linearity of the Frank-Starling relationship in the intact heart: the concept of preload recruitable stroke work. Circulation 1985;71(5):994–1009.

16. Kass DA, Beyar R. Evaluation of contractile state by maximal ventricular power divided by the square of end-diastolic volume. Circulation 1991;84(4): 1698–708.

17. Sharir T, Feldman MD, Haber H, et al. Ventricular systolic assessment in patients with dilated cardiomyopathy by preload-adjusted maximal power. Validation and noninvasive application. Circulation 1994;89(5):2045–53.

18. Senzaki H, Fetics B, Chen CH, et al. Comparison of ventricular pressure relaxation assessments in human heart failure: quantitative influence on load and drug sensitivity analysis. J Am Coll Cardiol 1999;34(5):1529–36.

19. Matsubara H, Takaki M, Yasuhara S, et al. Logistic time constant of isovolumic relaxation pressure-time curve in the canine left ventricle. Better alternative to exponential time constant. Circulation 1995; 92(8):2318–26.

20. Chung CS, Kovacs SJ. Physical determinants of left ventricular isovolumic pressure decline: model prediction with in vivo validation. Am J Physiol Heart Circ Physiol 2008;294(4):H1589–96.

21. Redfield MM, Jacobsen SJ, Burnett JC Jr, et al. Burden of systolic and diastolic ventricular dysfunction in the community: appreciating the scope of the heart failure epidemic. JAMA 2003;289(2):194–202.

22. Glantz SA, Parmley WW. Factors which affect the diastolic pressure-volume curve. Circ Res 1978; 42(2):171–80.

23. Oh JK, Hatle L, Tajik AJ, et al. Diastolic heart failure can be diagnosed by comprehensive two-dimensional and Doppler echocardiography. J Am Coll Cardiol 2006;47(3):500–6.

24. Kass DA. Assessment of diastolic dysfunction. Invasive modalities. Cardiol Clin 2000;18(3):571–86.

25. Pak PH, Maughan L, Baughman KL, et al. Marked discordance between dynamic and passive diastolic pressure-volume relations in idiopathic hypertrophic cardiomyopathy. Circulation 1996;94(1):52–60.

26. Zile MR, Baicu CF, Gaasch WH. Diastolic heart failure–abnormalities in active relaxation and passive stiffness of the left ventricle. N Engl J Med 2004;350(19):1953–9.

27. Westermann D, Kasner M, Steendijk P, et al. Role of left ventricular stiffness in heart failure with normal ejection fraction. Circulation 2008;117(16):2051–60.

28. Maurer MS, Burkhoff D, Fried LP, et al. Ventricular structure and function in hypertensive participants with heart failure and a normal ejection fraction: the Cardiovascular Health Study. J Am Coll Cardiol 2007;49(9):972–81.

29. Melenovsky V, Borlaug BA, Rosen B, et al. Cardiovascular features of heart failure with preserved ejection fraction versus nonfailing hypertensive left ventricular hypertrophy in the urban Baltimore community: the role of atrial remodeling/dysfunction. J Am Coll Cardiol 2007;49(2):198–207.

30. Dauterman K, Pak PH, Maughan WL, et al. Contribution of external forces to left ventricular diastolic pressure. Implications for the clinical use of the Starling law. Ann Intern Med 1995;122(10):737–42.

31. Frenneaux M, Williams L. Ventricular-arterial and ventricular-ventricular interactions and their relevance to diastolic filling. Prog Cardiovasc Dis 2007;49(4):252–62.

32. Kawaguchi M, Hay I, Fetics B, et al. Combined ventricular systolic and arterial stiffening in patients with heart failure and preserved ejection fraction: implications for systolic and diastolic reserve limitations. Circulation 2003;107(5):714–20.

33. Atherton JJ, Moore TD, Lele SS, et al. Diastolic ventricular interaction in chronic heart failure. Lancet 1997;349(9067):1720–4.

34. Moore TD, Frenneaux MP, Sas R, et al. Ventricular interaction and external constraint account for decreased stroke work during volume loading in CHF. Am J Physiol Heart Circ Physiol 2001;281(6): H2385–91.

35. Kass DA, Kelly RP. Ventriculo-arterial coupling: concepts, assumptions, and applications. Ann Biomed Eng 1992;20(1):41–62.

36. Milnor WR. Arterial impedance as ventricular afterload. Circ Res 1975;36(5):565–70.

37. Murgo JP, Westerhof N, Giolma JP, et al. Aortic input impedance in normal man: relationship to pressure wave forms. Circulation 1980;62(1):105–16.

38. Sunagawa K, Maughan WL, Burkhoff D, et al. Left ventricular interaction with arterial load studied in isolated canine ventricle. Am J Physiol 1983; 245(5 Pt 1):H773–80.

39. Sunagawa K, Maughan WL, Sagawa K. Optimal arterial resistance for the maximal stroke work studied in isolated canine left ventricle. Circ Res 1985;56(4):586–95.

40. Kelly RP, Ting CT, Yang TM, et al. Effective arterial elastance as index of arterial vascular load in humans. Circulation 1992;86(2):513–21.

41. De Tombe PP, Jones S, Burkhoff D, et al. Ventricular stroke work and efficiency both remain nearly optimal despite altered vascular loading. Am J Physiol 1993;264(6 Pt 2):H1817–24.

42. Asanoi H, Sasayama S, Kameyama T. Ventriculoarterial coupling in normal and failing heart in humans. Circ Res 1989;65(2):483–93.

43. Borlaug BA, Melenovsky V, Redfield MM, et al. Impact of arterial load and loading sequence on

left ventricular tissue velocities in humans. J Am Coll Cardiol 2007;50(16):1570–7.

44. Gillebert TC, Leite-Moreira AF, De Hert SG. Load dependent diastolic dysfunction in heart failure. Heart Fail Rev 2000;5(4):345–55.

45. Bilchick KC, Duncan JG, Ravi R, et al. Heart failure-associated alterations in troponin I phosphorylation impair ventricular relaxation-afterload and force-frequency responses and systolic function. Am J Physiol Heart Circ Physiol 2007;292(1):H318–25.

46. Shapiro BP, Lam CS, Patel JB, et al. Acute and chronic ventricular-arterial coupling in systole and diastole. Insights from an elderly hypertensive model. Hypertension 2007;50(3):503–11.

47. Haddad F, Doyle R, Murphy DJ, et al. Right ventricular function in cardiovascular disease, part II: pathophysiology, clinical importance, and management of right ventricular failure. Circulation 2008;117(13): 1717–31.

48. Kjaergaard J, Akkan D, Iversen KK, et al. Prognostic importance of pulmonary hypertension in patients with heart failure. Am J Cardiol 2007;99(8):1146–50.

49. McGoon M, Gutterman D, Steen V, et al. Screening, early detection, and diagnosis of pulmonary arterial hypertension: ACCP evidence-based clinical practice guidelines. Chest 2004;126(1 Suppl):14S–34S.

50. Alaeddini J, Uber PA, Park MH, et al. Efficacy and safety of sildenafil in the evaluation of pulmonary hypertension in severe heart failure. Am J Cardiol 2004;94(11):1475–7.

51. Shapiro BP, McGoon MD, Redfield MM. Unexplained pulmonary hypertension in elderly patients. Chest 2007;131(1):94–100.

52. Kussmaul WG 3rd, Altschuler JA, Matthai WH, et al. Right ventricular-vascular interaction in congestive heart failure. Importance of low-frequency impedance. Circulation 1993;88(3):1010–5.

53. Lepore JJ, Maroo A, Bigatello LM, et al. Hemodynamic effects of sildenafil in patients with congestive heart failure and pulmonary hypertension: combined administration with inhaled nitric oxide. Chest 2005; 127(5):1647–53.

54. Lewis GD, Lachmann J, Camuso J, et al. Sildenafil improves exercise hemodynamics and oxygen uptake in patients with systolic heart failure. Circulation 2007;115(1):59–66.

55. Guazzi M, Samaja M, Arena R, et al. Long-term use of sildenafil in the therapeutic management of heart failure. J Am Coll Cardiol 2007;50(22):2136–44.

56. Costello-Boerrigter LC, Boerrigter G, Redfield MM, et al. Amino-terminal pro-B-type natriuretic peptide and B-type natriuretic peptide in the general community: determinants and detection of left ventricular dysfunction. J Am Coll Cardiol 2006; 47(2):345–53.

57. Hurrell DG, Nishimura RA, Higano ST, et al. Value of dynamic respiratory changes in left and right ventricular pressures for the diagnosis of constrictive pericarditis. Circulation 1996;93(11):2007–13.

58. Talreja DR, Nishimura RA, Oh JK, et al. Constrictive pericarditis in the modern era: novel criteria for diagnosis in the cardiac catheterization laboratory. J Am Coll Cardiol 2008;51(3):315–9.

59. Suga H, Sagawa K, Demer L. Determinants of instantaneous pressure in canine left ventricle. Time and volume specification. Circ Res 1980; 46(2):256–63.

60. Kass DA, Solaro RJ. Mechanisms and use of calcium-sensitizing agents in the failing heart. Circulation 2006;113(2):305–15.

Are Hemodynamic Parameters Predictors of Mortality?

Garrie J. Haas, MD*, Carl V. Leier, MD

KEYWORDS

- Decompensated heart failure • Congestion
- Hemodynamics • Heart failure pathophysiology • Mortality

The heart failure (HF) syndrome is a common and complex condition associated with significant mortality. Over the past 2 decades, despite important advances in pharmacotherapy and devices, hospital admissions for HF have risen more than 150% and represent the most common reason for hospitalization in persons over 65 years of age.[1,2] Clinical decompensation is a critical event for the patient who has HF and has major prognostic implications including significant mortality. A seeming paradox is that although most patients do not die during the index hospitalization (mortality averages 5%–8%), there is a 10% risk of death in the ensuing 60 to 90 days, and the 1-year mortality following an acute HF exacerbation approaches 35%.[2–5] Ahmed and colleagues,[6] reviewing data from the Digitalis Investigation Group trial, found that incident hospitalization is associated with significant subsequent mortality compared with those with no prior hospitalization for HF (hazards ratio [HR] 2.49, 95% confidence interval [CI], 1.97–3.13; $P < .0001$). A recent post hoc analysis of the Candesartan in Heart Failure Assessment of Reduction in Mortality and Morbidity (CHARM) database demonstrated similar findings: HF hospitalization was independently associated with increased mortality (HR, 3.15; 95% CI, 2.83–3.50; $P = .0001$).[7] The reason for this dramatic impact of hospitalization on the natural history of HF has not been elucidated but is the focus of ongoing clinical investigation. One hypothesis, related to the current topic, is that congestion (and consequently abnormal hemodynamics) persists in some patients despite clinical improvement during the hospitalization.[8]

Because HF represents a progressive condition that is a manifestation of the interplay of multiple pathobiologic perturbations, the identification of specific factors associated with a poor prognosis that may represent viable therapeutic targets has been challenging. The list of predictors of increased mortality has grown exponentially in recent years in concert with the improved understanding of the HF syndrome and its various clinical manifestations during disease progression.[9] Several predictive algorithms have been created to assist the clinician in risk assessment for the individual patient, particularly when considering referral for advanced therapies such as cardiac transplantation or mechanical support.[10–16] Unfortunately, with the exception of those few patients who go on to receive a cardiac transplant or a left ventricular assist device (LVAD), knowledge of the specific mortality risk for the individual does not necessarily alter therapy or translate to improved outcomes. The question therefore may be asked whether mortality prediction really is helpful in the majority of patients who are not yet candidates for transplantation, given the current recommendation, that certain therapies (angiotensin-converting enzyme inhibitors, beta-blockers, aldosterone antagonists) always must be used.

To address this issue, one must consider that although a relatively strong evidence base exists for patients who have chronic, stable HF, the same does not apply to those at greatest risk for

The Ohio State University Medical Center, Columbus, OH, USA

* Corresponding author. Division of Cardiovascular Medicine, Department of Internal Medicine, The Ohio State University Medical Center, Suite 200, Davis Heart/Lung Institute, 473 W. 12th Avenue, Columbus, OH 43210.

E-mail address: garrie.haas@osumc.edu (G.J. Haas).

Heart Failure Clin 5 (2009) 229–240
doi:10.1016/j.hfc.2008.11.007
1551-7136/08/$ – see front matter © 2009 Elsevier Inc. All rights reserved.

death, specifically patients who have recent or ongoing decompensation.[2,17-19] In this HF cohort therapeutic approaches beyond the current evidence base often are necessary for symptom relief with the expectation for improved outcomes. Although, given the current relevance of neurohormonal antagonism, many clinicians may consider the focus on the hemodynamic paradigm obsolete, the authors of this article believe that in the high-risk subgroup of patients who have decompensated HF, hemodynamic derangement is a consistent finding, is prognostically important, and is linked closely to symptoms, disease progression, and survival. Although yet to be proven in randomized trials, tailoring therapy to hemodynamic targets may be even more valid in the current era of HF management, when novel direct and indirect methods for monitoring hemodynamics are available clinically or are being investigated.[20,21] Furthermore, it is clear that merely ensuring the introduction of evidence-based therapies at the time of hospital discharge does not guarantee freedom from early rehospitalization or death.[22]

This article addresses a question that the authors consider to be somewhat rhetorical: "Are hemodynamic parameters predictors of mortality?" The specific hemodynamic abnormalities and pathophysiologic consequences distinctive to the patient who has decompensation are reviewed. The data that implicate abnormal hemodynamics as a treatment target associated with increased mortality are addressed. The focus is on patients who have decompensated HF, defined as left ventricular systolic dysfunction and an acute, subacute, or gradual worsening of symptoms while receiving optimal medical therapy.[2,4] This subgroup of patients who have HF represents those who have disease progression despite therapies designed to prevent or delay HF evolution. This subgroup is representative of the HF population in which the association between hemodynamic derangement and mortality is most evident and in whom "tailored therapy" to a specific hemodynamic target may be most pertinent.[20,23-25]

THE HEMODYNAMICS OF DECOMPENSATION

HF decompensation in a patient who has previously stable, chronic HF represents approximately 75% to 80% of all hospitalizations for HF according to large international registries.[26-29] These patients, despite optimal medical therapy in the outpatient setting, often have reduced functional capacity on a chronic basis and may have some degree of volume overload, even when perceived to be clinically compensated. Left ventricular wall stress, because of left ventricular dilatation, usually is elevated, and "compensatory" neurohormonal mechanisms are heavily involved.[2] When decompensation occurs, leading to hospitalization, clinical findings of congestion usually are readily apparent. The most common congestive findings and frequency of occurrence according to the Acute Decompensated Heart Failure National Registry (ADHERE) database are dyspnea and dyspnea at rest (90% and 34%, respectively), pulmonary rales (67%), and peripheral edema (66%).[26] The decompensation process, which may occur over days to weeks, is associated with progressive hemodynamic deterioration manifest primarily as an increase in left ventricular filling pressure (LVFP) and secondary pulmonary hypertension. In the Vasodilation in the Management of Congestive Heart Failure trial,[30] those admitted for decompensated HF in whom invasive hemodynamic monitoring was performed with pulmonary artery catheterization (PAC) had a pulmonary capillary wedge pressure (PCWP) of 25 to 30 mm Hg but preserved cardiac output. The PCWP, in the absence of mitral stenosis or pulmonary venous disease, generally correlates well with the LVFP. In HF there are several possible reasons for elevated LVFP, including sodium and medication noncompliance. High LVFPs, often a consequence of worsening left ventricular function regardless of cause, underlie most of the symptoms observed on presentation.

It is recognized that specific clinical conditions often associated with decompensated HF, such as atrial fibrillation, myocardial ischemia, and hypertension, result in elevated LVFP. As stated earlier, this process may occur gradually without an immediate change in symptomatology and in most cases results from volume or pressure overload with fluid redistribution to the pulmonary vasculature.[31] Unfortunately, the sensitivity of congestive symptoms as a predictor or warning of high LVFP is poor. In other words, the "absence" of symptoms or physical findings does not guarantee that LVFP is optimal. Several studies have evaluated the sensitivity of symptoms, physical findings, or chest radiographs to predict increased PCWP, concluding that signs and symptoms have a relatively poor predictive value for identifying patients who have a PCWP higher than 30 mm Hg. In a study by Mahdyoon and colleagues,[32] only 7 of 22 patients (32%) who had an elevated PCWP had chest radiographic findings consistent with pulmonary venous hypertension or congestion. In another study, clinical signs had only a 58% sensitivity in detecting patients who had a significant elevation in LVFP (or PCWP).[33] In the recently reported Efficacy of Vasopressin Antagonism in Heart Failure Outcome Study with Tolvaptan trial, only 27% of patients reportedly had jugular venous distension greater than 10 cm in a populations of congested patients who had advanced HF.[34] These observations that patients who have congestion may be difficult to recognize on routine clinical assessment has popularized the term "hemodynamic congestion," which basically represents a state of elevated LVFP without evidence of clinical congestion.[21] Although clinical congestion usually is a late finding that often precipitates the hospitalization, hemodynamic congestion may persist for an extended period in the absence of clinical signs or symptoms. This concept identifies two points on a continuum in the development of congestion, and the awareness of this continuum may allow the clinician to intervene earlier and prevent hospitalization and its important prognostic implications.[21] Although signs and symptoms of congestion are helpful if recognized, the absence of clinical findings cannot assure the clinician of optimal hemodynamics.

Traditional methods for detecting hemodynamic congestion and impending hospitalization, such as daily weights and monitoring fluid intake and output, in addition to clinical assessment, also are often unreliable. It has been shown that monitoring daily weights and symptoms does not consistently reduce hospitalization for patients who have moderate to severe HF.[35,36] Most patients report dyspnea only hours to days before hospitalization. This experience is in marked contrast to the findings from more recent trials evaluating more sensitive and accurate measurements of LVFP, such as implantable hemodynamic monitoring devices and intrathoracic impedance monitors.[36,37] A growing experience with these devices has shown that hemodynamic congestion may occur days to weeks in advance of clinical decompensation. These methodologies may provide the clinician with an opportunity for early intervention to prevent decompensated HF. This concept is addressed in detail elsewhere in this issue.

CONSEQUENCES OF ELEVATED LEFT VENTRICULAR FILLING PRESSURE

A sustained elevation in LVFP is a marker of disease progression and contributes significantly to the pathologic process. An elevated LVFP may affect left ventricular remodeling directly and, if it remains untreated, may accelerate the natural history of the disease. In fact, it has been hypothesized that the failure to improve LVFP adequately

during a hospitalization may account in part for subsequent readmissions for decompensated HF.[8,21] A large percentage of those admitted who have decompensated HF may not experience meaningful weight loss (volume reduction) during the hospitalization. The ADHERE registry data indicate that, despite the use of diuretics in 88% of hospitalized patients who have decompensated HF, as many as 20% have no weight loss or even have weight gain by the time of discharge.[26,27] Given the known lack of connection between clinical findings and hemodynamic congestion, it is conceivable that these patients may be discharged from the hospital with persistent elevation of LVFP, only to experience a recurrence of symptoms at a later date. This important association was observed in the recently reported Evaluation Study of Congestive Heart Failure and Pulmonary Artery Catheter Effectiveness (ESCAPE) trial. Patients who had persistent elevation in filling pressures during treatment (as measured with PAC) were most likely to have symptoms or reduced functional capacity at 3 months after hospital discharge (**Fig. 1**).[20,38]

A chronic elevation in LVFP results in a cascade of detrimental hemodynamic, neuroendocrine, and inflammatory effects that perpetuate the cardiac-remodeling process that includes ventricular dilation and increased sphericity, eccentric hypertrophy, and interstitial fibrosis.[39] Elevated LVFP, directly and/or via cellular signaling

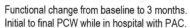
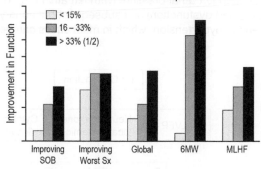

Fig. 1. Relationship of reduction in pulmonary capillary wedge pressures (PCW) during hospitalization to improvement in symptoms (Sx) measured at 3 months after hospital discharge, from the ESCAPE trial. Average PCW (measured with pulmonary artery catheter, PAC) decreased from 25 mm Hg to 17 mm Hg during monitoring, and more than half of the patients had a greater than 33% reduction in PCW. MLHF, Minnesota Living with Heart Failure questionnaire; SOB, shortness of breath; 6MW, 6-minute walk. (*From* Stevenson LW. Hemodynamic goals are relevant. Circulation 2006;113:1021; with permission.)

processes, contributes to increased wall stress and ventricular dilatation. Accompanying contributing factors include maladaptive neurohormonal responses leading to activation of the renin-angiotensin-aldosterone system, sympathetic nervous system, arginine vasopressin, endothelin, elevation of inflammatory cytokines, reduced nitric oxide production, continued sodium and water retention, and potent vascular constricting effects, all promoting an increase in ventricular load.[2,40–43] In fact, increased filling pressures and myocardial stretch are among the most powerful mechanisms causing neurohormonal activation as well as the activation of adverse gene expression programs and induction of myocyte apoptosis.[43] Structural changes including dilation and change in the shape of the left ventricle from elliptic to spherical results in increased myocardial oxygen demand, atrioventricular valve insufficiency, and compromised stroke volume.[41–43] Because of elevated LVFP, myocardial and interstitial edema, and a tachycardia-related reduction in diastolic perfusion time, subendocardial perfusion is compromised, and myocardial ischemia may occur. This process probably accounts for elevated troponin levels, despite normal coronary arteries, in patients who have advanced HF.[42] Thus, a vicious cycle of deterioration is generated and perpetuated as a result of elevated LVFP and volume overload. This pathophysiologic process forms much of the rationale that relates abnormal hemodynamic parameters to mortality.

Even in the absence of intrinsic mitral valve disease, a chronic elevation in LVFP results in elevated left atrial pressure (with left atrial remodeling and dysfunction) and subsequent pulmonary venous hypertension, which in most cases can be considered a consequence of high filling pressures.[31] In most patients, this process results in pulmonary artery hypertension which usually is reversible with diuretic and vasoactive therapy. If these hemodynamic abnormalities persist, however, right-sided pressure and volume overload ultimately occur. In the most chronic and severe cases, sustained pulmonary venous hypertension may result in severe pulmonary artery hypertension (systolic pulmonary artery pressures as high as 80 mm Hg) with pathologic remodeling of the pulmonary vasculature, a process similar to that seen in chronic severe mitral stenosis or idiopathic pulmonary hypertension (**Fig. 2**).[44] In these patients, the risk of developing right heart failure is substantial and is associated with poor survival (**Fig. 3**).[44–46] When the disease has advanced to this degree, the transpulmonic gradient (the mean pulmonary artery pressure minus the PCWP) often is increased, and acute vasodilator challenge, despite reducing LVFP, does not reverse the pulmonary hypertension readily. This ominous finding of "fixed" pulmonary hypertension must be routinely excluded in those awaiting cardiac transplantation. The inability to lower pulmonary pressures adequately by manipulating the left ventricular load is an absolute contraindication to cardiac transplantation and remains the most common reason for the acute early postoperative failure of the transplanted allograft.[47–49]

In the past, decompensated HF often was viewed as a disorder of low cardiac output, but for the reasons outlined earlier in this article and because of the observations made from large registries, therapy focussed on LVFP has taken precedence. Although a compromised cardiac output may have set the process in motion, the

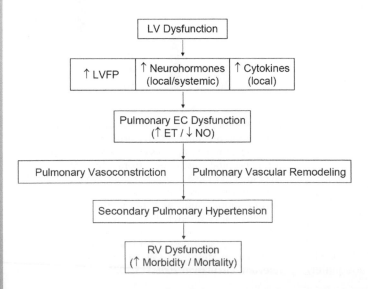

Fig. 2. Proposed relationship between left ventricular dysfunction and secondary events that may contribute to development of pulmonary hypertension. ET, endothelin; LV, left ventricle; LVFP, left ventricular filling pressure; NO, nitric oxide; RV, right ventricle. (*From* Moraes DL, Colucci WS, Givertz MM. Secondary pulmonary hypertension in chronic heart failure. The role of the endothelium in pathophysiology and management. Circulation 2000;102:1719; with permission.)

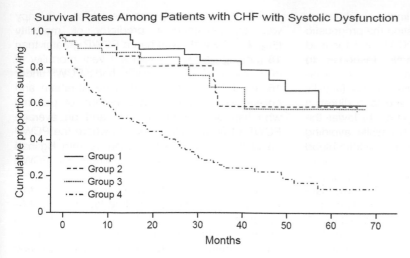

Survival Rates Among Patients with CHF with Systolic Dysfunction

Fig. 3. Survival rates among patients who have heart failure are significantly worse in those who have elevated pulmonary artery pressure (PAP) and reduced right ventricular ejection fraction (RVEF). Group 1: normal PAP, preserved RVEF (n = 73). Group 2: normal PAP, low RVEF (n = 68). Group 3: high PAP, preserved RVEF (n = 21). Group 4: high PAP, low RVEF (n = 215). CHF, chronic heart failure. (*From* Ghio S, Gavazzi A, Campana C, et al. Independent and additive prognostic value of right ventricular systolic function and pulmonary artery pressure in patients with chronic heart failure. J Am Coll Cardiol 2001;37:187; with permission.)

persistence of a high LVFP fuels detrimental ventricular remodeling and symptoms. Most patients admitted to the hospital with decompensation do not have an inordinately low cardiac output. Also, pharmacologic measures to enhance cardiac output acutely have not improved outcomes and even may increase mortality.[2,4]

It has been proposed that failure to improve cardiac output and renal perfusion underlies the common problem of renal dysfunction in HF. It is known that even very small decrements in renal function during HF management predict increased mortality.[50–52] A recent study by Nohria and colleagues,[52] however, did not identify poor cardiac output or renal hypoperfusion as a cause of worsening renal function in decompensated HF. It is likely that the etiology of kidney disease in HF results from a combination of disturbances and cannot be isolated to merely one abnormality. For example, it has been known for years that the relationship between hemodynamics and renal responses are abnormal in HF.[53] In response to an elevation in left atrial pressure, the atrial–renal reflexes that normally enhance sodium and water excretion are blunted and dysfunctional in HF, resulting in the tendency to retain sodium and water.[21,54] In addition, information now available links intra-abdominal congestion and abdominal and renal venous pressure with the renal dysfunction of HF.[55] These findings highlight the multisystem nature and inherent complexity of the HF syndrome; thus it is naïve to expect that a single variable will be identified that will impact prognosis significantly. The challenge is to identify and address all treatable factors that cumulatively impact morbidity and mortality.

HEMODYNAMICS AND PROGNOSIS

Considering the detrimental effect of elevated filling pressures on ventricular remodeling and disease progression, it is to be expected that LVFP and related parameters (jugular venous pressure, natriuretic peptides, persistent symptoms) are linked robustly to mortality.[20,56–60] Over the past 20 years, a series of clinical observations, using PAC to measure PCWP and estimate LVFP, have identified a clear association between LVFP and mortality. Early studies reported by Unverferth and colleagues,[56] Franciosa and colleagues,[57] and others identified abnormal baseline hemodynamics as predictive of survival in patients with a broad spectrum of disease severity and therapies.[58–60] In the current era of HF management, despite improvement in overall survival for patients who have advanced HF on cardiac transplant waiting lists, a PCWP higher than 20 mm Hg has remained one of the predictors of death within 2 months of listing.[58]

Much of the knowledge concerning the importance of LVFP, its relationship to survival, and its potential as a treatment target comes from the seminal work of Stevenson and colleagues[20,21,23–25] beginning with observations made in the late 1980s. These investigators introduced the concept of tailored therapy targeted to normalize the PCWP to improve symptoms and predict outcomes. Contrary to prior studies that had used a percent reduction in PCWP during treatment, these investigators sought to "normalize" the PCWP with aggressive vasodilator, diuretic, and angiotensin-converting enzyme inhibitor therapy with the hypothesis that achieving normal hemodynamics would improve outcomes. Their results brought into question the prognostic implications of the baseline PCWP and focused attention on the hemodynamic response to optimal therapy. The approach involved administration of intravenous vasoactive therapy (usually nitroprusside or nitroglycerin) and loop diuretics during PAC monitoring in an effort to lower the PCWP to less than 16 mm Hg while avoiding systemic hypotension (maintaining systolic blood pressure above 80 mm Hg).[61] When these goals were accomplished, transition to oral therapy to sustain the observed reduction in PCWP was instituted while continuing to monitor hemodynamics. When the hemodynamic goals were achieved, the difference in mortality observed over the short term between responders and nonresponders was remarkable. This tailored approach was tested in 152 patients who had advanced HF and a baseline PCWP of 28 mm Hg who were referred to their tertiary care center for cardiac transplantation.[24] Patients exhibiting a favorable response to vasoactive treatment with lowering of the PCWP to target levels (< 16 mm Hg) had a 1-year survival of 83%, compared with 38% for those who were considered nonresponders. In a similar study, these same investigators found that failure to achieve a target PCWP despite titration of

angiotensin-converting enzyme inhibitor therapy was an independent predictor of mortality (**Fig. 4**).[59] Patients who had a PCWP greater than 18 mm Hg on therapy had a 1-year mortality of 36%, versus 18% in those who had a PCWP under 16 mm Hg. A study reported by Abraham and colleagues[59] evaluated two groups of patients who had decompensated HF and an average PCWP of 30 mm Hg. Those in whom the PCWP could be reduced to less than 16 mm Hg had half the mortality of those in whom the PCWP could not be lowered to this level. A lower PCWP achieved during treatment in the ESCAPE trial also identified patients who had lower rates of 6-month events.[20,38] In all these studies, changes in cardiac output did not seem to predict survival, and the central hemodynamic response to therapy was much more pertinent even than baseline LVFP. Thus, these and a host of similar findings from direct assessment of LVFP with PAC during HF hospitalization have supported the notion that a reduction in LVFP during management is an important prognostic finding and goal of therapy. In patients who have advanced disease whose LVFP cannot be lowered despite aggressive pharmacologic manipulation, the prognosis is poor, and therapeutic options including cardiac transplantation and/or LVAD should be explored. It

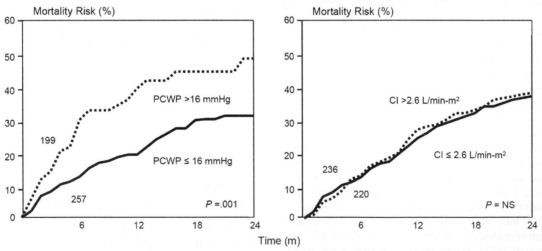

Fig. 4. The failure to reduce pulmonary capillary wedge pressure (PCWP) during tailored therapy, including high-dose angiotensin-converting enzyme inhibitors, identified patients who had HF and who had significant mortality risk. High PCWP on aggressive therapy was an independent predictor of overall mortality in these 456 patients who had advanced heart failure. Although the change in PCWP during therapy was relevant, the cardiac index (CI) did not predict subsequent mortality. (*From* Fonarow GC, Stevenson LW, Steimle AE, et al. Persistently high left ventricular filling pressures predict mortality despite angiotensin converting enzyme inhibition in advanced heart failure. Circulation 1994;90:I-488; with permission.)

follows, therefore, that hemodynamic parameters, in this instance LVFP and changes thereof, are linked to mortality.

Although these data are compelling and certainly link LVFP and mortality in patients who have HF, it remains to be determined whether a strategy to treat elevated LVFP actually creates survivors or merely identifies them.[20,43,61] One could argue that the actual process of lowering pressures is not pertinent, but the ability to do so simply identifies patients with better cardiac reserve, less advanced disease, and thus better outcomes. Considering the multiplicity of adverse effects of high LVFP on cardiac anatomy and function, neuroendocrine response, and peripheral vascular effects, as described previously, it seems likely that a direct relationship exists between LVFP and outcomes, and the treatment effect on LVFP is contributory.

Future studies using implantable hemodynamic monitoring systems probably will add important insight into the role and merit of treating high LVFP to improve outcomes in HF. In a subgroup of patients in the recently reported randomized, controlled, single-blind Chronicle Offers Management to Patients With Advanced Signs and Symptoms of Heart Failure trial, therapy based on continuous hemodynamic monitoring reduced first HF-related hospitalizations by 36%.[62] In another study using continuous hemodynamic monitoring, adjustment of HF therapy to maintain the estimated LVFP below 22 mm Hg was associated with a highly significant reduction in HF events.[63] Additional research using both invasive and noninvasive hemodynamic monitoring systems is currently underway.

HEMODYNAMIC SURROGATES AND PROGNOSIS

Because results from the ESCAPE trial did not favor therapy guided by hemodynamic monitoring over that guided by signs and symptoms of HF during hospitalization, the routine use of PAC to direct treatment cannot be recommended for hospitalized patients who have advanced HF. Because most patients admitted to the hospital who have decompensated HF are congested and symptomatic, it is not surprising that symptom-directed therapy may be effective in most otherwise uncomplicated patients. The authors believe that this finding does not dilute the importance of hemodynamic goals during hospitalization, because most symptoms and HF therapies are related to elevated filling pressures. Furthermore, the clinician's ability to assess and respond to abnormal hemodynamics, without invasive monitoring and use of PAC, has been advanced in recent years by various surrogate hemodynamic parameters, several of which are discussed briefly here.

The basic signs and symptoms of congestion are reasonably specific for predicting an elevation in LVFP, but, as previously mentioned, their sensitivity is poor and is dependent on the experience of the clinician.[64] Elevated jugular venous pressure and a third heart sound, both reflecting high LVFP, are known to correlate with adverse events.[65,66] Right atrial pressure greater than 10 mm Hg has been shown to track with PCWPs greater than 22 mm Hg in approximately 80% of patients who have chronic HF.[66] Lucas and colleagues[67] found that clinical evidence of congestion 4 to 6 weeks following a hospitalization for HF identified patients at high risk for decompensation (**Fig. 5**). These investigators used common clinical criteria including weight change, jugular venous pressure, orthopnea, edema, and need for increased diuretics. Therefore, if these findings are present in an individual patient, they are therapeutically and prognostically important. More often, however, they are not recognized with confidence, and, importantly, their absence does not exclude elevated LVFP and pulmonary congestion.

Measurement of the plasma levels of B-type natriuretic peptide (BNP) is a relatively sensitive and specific test for elevated LVFP. BNP is released from the left ventricle in response to elevated filling pressures and increased wall stress

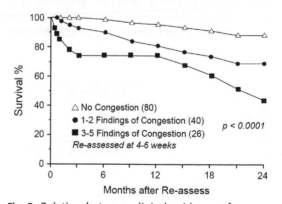

Fig. 5. Relation between clinical evidence of congestion (orthopnea, weight gain, jugular venous pressure, increased diuretic use, peripheral edema) at 4 to 6 weeks after hospitalization and survival over subsequent 2 years for 146 patients who had decompensated heart failure. (*From* Lucas C, Johnson W, Hamilton MA, et al. Freedom from congestion predicts good survival despite previous class IV symptoms of heart failure. Am Heart J 2000;140:843; with permission.)

and has been shown to track changes in PCWP relatively closely.[68] In the ADHERE registry, the median BNP level was 840 pg/mL at the time of hospitalization for HF.[4] Evidence continues to mount showing that BNP also is predictive of mortality in chronic HF.[68] It has been estimated that every 100-pg/mL increase in BNP is associated with a 35% increase in the risk of death.[69] Analogous to the predictive value of a treatment-related reduction in PCWP, a low predischarge BNP level also has been identified as a marker for improved outcomes.[70] The failure to observe a substantive reduction in BNP during hospitalization and treatment for HF identifies patients who are at increased risk of death or rehospitalization. Logeart and colleagues[70] reported that the risk of death or rehospitalization increased in step-wise fashion across increasing predischarge BNP ranges (**Fig. 6**). Remarkably, the HR for patients who had persistent elevation of BNP (> 700 ng/L) was 15.2 (95% CI, 8.5–27) compared with those who had a predischarge BNP of less than 350 ng/L. Results from a recent multicenter study to evaluate the prognostic impact of a therapeutic strategy guided by plasma BNP levels in the outpatient setting are pertinent.[71] BNP-guided adjustments in evidence-based therapy significantly reduced the risk of HF-related death or hospital stay compared with standard outpatient care. This finding further emphasizes the risk of failure to identify and respond to "hemodynamic" congestion. In this trial, the elevated BNP served as a stimulus for the clinician to increase further the dosing of important medications, including angiotensin-converting enzyme inhibitors and beta-blockers, when otherwise they would not have been adjusted based on clinical findings

alone. In a recently reported retrospective study of 186 patients who had decompensated HF, the patients who had predischarge BNP levels less than 250 pg/mL exhibited a 6-month event rate of 16%, compared with 78% in those who had higher BNP levels at discharge.[72] The totality of the BNP data further supports the construct that high LVFP is linked to rehospitalization and mortality and that significant reversal of LVFP identifies those who have improved outcomes.

Echocardiography provides a reasonably accurate and safe means for rapidly assessing central hemodynamics in patients who have HF. An echocardiography/Doppler-based strategy for tailoring HF therapy has been described.[73] Rohde and colleagues[74] used echocardiography and Doppler-based estimates of hemodynamic parameters, or clinical evaluation alone, to guide treatment in 96 outpatients who had HF. Survival at 230 days was significantly better when echocardiography was used to guide therapy. Importantly, this group had a treatment-related improvement in pulmonary artery pressures and received higher doses of vasodilators (hydralazine) and diuretics. These results are consistent with those reported by Ristow and colleagues,[75] who found that Doppler estimates of pulmonary artery systolic and diastolic pressure were predictive of hospitalization for HF or death.

Thus, a number of methodologies currently are available to assist the clinician in evaluating hemodynamics without the need and associated morbidity of invasive monitoring with PAC. From the data presented, the information derived from these methods also supports a strong association between hemodynamic abnormalities and major outcomes in HF.

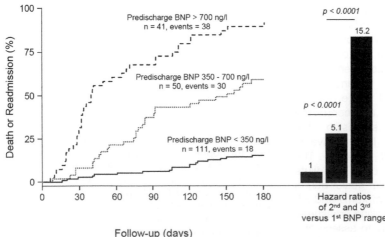

Fig. 6. Kaplan-Meier curves showing the cumulative incidence of death or rehospitalization according to predischarge B-type natriuretic peptide (BNP) ranges (< 350, 350–700, or > 700 ng/L) in 105 patients who had decompensated HF. High predischarge BNP was a strong, independent marker of death or re-admission. Hazard ratios are shown for each BNP range. (*From* Logeart D, Thabut G, Jourdain P, et al. Predischarge B-type natriuretic peptide assay for identifying patients at high risk for readmission after decompensated heart failure. J Am Coll Cardiol 2004;43:639; with permission.)

MECHANICAL VENTRICULAR UNLOADING AND PROGNOSIS

The reversal of ventricular remodeling by unloading the ventricle with LVAD support is perhaps the most extreme example of the potential benefit derived from reducing LVFP. Sustained normalization of LVFP, even in patients who have advanced HF requiring mechanical support, has been found to contribute to recovery of left ventricular function.[76] Although the reverse remodeling process is aided by aggressive medical therapy, a major requirement is complete unloading of the ventricle to allow myocardial recovery. This particular example supports the concept that the reversal of high LVFP directly impacts ventricular recovery and survival and is not just a marker that identifies patients who have better outcomes. The patients who exhibited recovery with LVAD would have had a poor prognosis otherwise, given their failure to respond to medical therapy.[77]

SUMMARY

Decompensated HF represents a complex condition associated with significant morbidity and mortality. Symptoms of congestion are common at the time of hospitalization and usually reflect elevated LVFP. It now is recognized that hemodynamic congestion and its detrimental pathobiologic consequences may exist well in advance of symptom development and also may persist after symptom resolution. This problem of incompletely treated and clinically unrecognized hemodynamic congestion may account for the substantial morbidity and mortality associated with HF hospitalizations. Although a strong association exists between both direct and surrogate markers of elevated LVFP and mortality in patients who have HF, it remains to be demonstrated whether tailored therapy directly affects outcomes or merely identifies those patients who have less advanced disease and better survival.

Multiple monitoring devices designed to assess cardiac filling pressures directly or indirectly and to guide therapy have been developed.[36,62,68,78-80] It is hoped that the results from studies using this technology will provide valuable insight regarding the role of more aggressive, hemodynamically directed therapy in the patients who have HF in which standard, evidence-based treatment has failed.

REFERENCES

1. Thom T, Haase N, Rosamond W, et al. Heart disease and stroke statistics—2006 update. A report from the American Heart Association Statistics Committee and the Stroke Statistics Subcommittee. Circulation 2006;113:e85–151.

2. Iyengar S, Haas GJ, Young JB. Acute heart failure. In: Topol EJ, editor. Textbook of cardiovascular medicine. 3rd edition. Philadelphia: Lippincott, Williams & Wilkins; 2007. p. 1352–72.

3. Kalon KL, Ho MD, Keaven M, et al. Survival after the onset of congestive heart failure in Framingham Heart Study subjects. Circulation 1993;88:107–15.

4. Fonarow GC. Acute decompensated heart failure: challenges and opportunities. Rev Cardiovasc Med 2007;8(Suppl 5):S3–12.

5. Jong P, Vowinckel E, Liu PP, et al. Prognosis and determinants of survival in patients newly hospitalized for heart failure. Arch Intern Med 2002;162:1689–94.

6. Ahmed A, Allman RM, Fonarow GC, et al. Incident heart failure hospitalization and subsequent mortality in chronic heart failure: a propensity-matched study. J Card Fail 2008;14:211–8.

7. Solomon SD, Dobson J, Pocock S, et al. Influence of nonfatal hospitalization for heart failure on subsequent mortality in patients with chronic heart failure. Circulation 2007;116:1482–7.

8. Costanzo MR, Guglin ME, Saltzberg MT, et al. Ultra-filtration versus intravenous diuretics for patients hospitalized for acute decompensated heart failure. J Am Coll Cardiol 2007;49:675–83.

9. Young JB. The prognosis of heart failure. In: Mann DL, editor. Heart failure: a companion to Braunwald's heart disease. 1st edition. Philadelphia: Saunders; 2004. p. 489–505.

10. Cleland JGF, Dargie HJ, Ford I. Mortality in heart failure: clinical variables of prognostic value. Br Heart J 1987;58:572–82.

11. Komajda M, Jais JP, Reeves F, et al. Factors predicting mortality in idiopathic dilated cardiomyopathy. Eur Heart J 1990;11:824–31.

12. Campana C, Gavazzi A, Berzuini C, et al. Predictors of prognosis in patients awaiting heart transplantation. J Heart Lung Transplant 1993;12:756–65.

13. Poses RM, Smith WR, McClish DK, et al. Physicians survival predictions for patients with acute congestive heart failure. Arch Intern Med 1997;157:1001–7.

14. Levy WC, Mozaffarian D, Linker DT, et al. The Seattle Heart Failure Model: prediction of survival in heart failure. Circulation 2006;113:1424–33.

15. Lee DS, Austin PC, Rouleau JL, et al. Predicting mortality among patients hospitalized for heart failure: derivation and validation of a clinical model. JAMA 2003;290:2581–7.

16. Aaronson KD, Schwartz JS, Chen TM, et al. Development and prospective validation of a clinical index to predict survival in ambulatory patients referred for cardiac transplant evaluation. Circulation 1997;95:2660–7.

17. Haas GJ, Abraham WT. Comprehensive pharmacologic management strategies in heart failure.

In: Yu CM, Hayes DL, Auricchio A, editors. Cardiac resynchronization therapy. Oxford (UK): Blackwell; 2008. p. 15–34.

18. Haas GJ, Abraham WT. The challenge of heart failure therapy: so many drugs, so little blood pressure. ACC Review 2005;10:36–40.

19. Hunt SA, Abraham WT, Chin MH, et al. ACC/AHA 2005 guideline update for the diagnosis and management of chronic heart failure in the adult: a report of the American College of Cardiology/American Heart Association task force on practice guidelines (Writing Committee to Update the 2001 guidelines for the evaluation and management of heart failure). Circulation 2005;112:1825–52.

20. Stevenson LW. Hemodynamic goals are relevant. Circulation 2006;113:1020–33.

21. Gheorghiade M, Filippatos G, De Luca L, et al. Congestion in acute heart failure syndromes: an essential target of evaluation and treatment. Am J Med 2006;119:S3–10.

22. Fonarow GC, Abraham WT, Albert NM, et al. Association between performance measures and clinical outcomes for patients hospitalized with heart failure. JAMA 2007;297:61–70.

23. Stevenson LW, Dracup KA, Tillisch JH. Efficacy of medical therapy tailored for severe congestive heart failure in patients transferred for urgent cardiac transplantation. Am J Cardiol 1989;63:461–4.

24. Stevenson LW, Tillisch JH, Hamilton M, et al. Importance of hemodynamic response to therapy in predicting survival with ejection fraction <20% secondary to ischemic or non-ischemic dilated cardiomyopathy. Am J Cardiol 1990;6:1348–54.

25. Stevenson LW. Tailored therapy before transplantation for treatment of advanced heart failure: effective use of vasodilators and diuretics. J Heart Lung Transplant 1991;10:468–76.

26. Fonarow GC, Heywood JT, Heidenreich PA, et al. Temporal trends in clinical characteristics, treatments, and outcomes for heart failure hospitalizations, 2002–2004: findings from Acute Decompensated Heart Failure National Registry (ADHERE). Am Heart J 2007;153:1021–8.

27. Adams KF, Fonarow GC, Emerman CL, et al. For the ADHERE Scientific Advisory Committee and Investigators. Characteristics and outcomes of patients hospitalized for heart failure in the United States: rationale, design, and preliminary observations from the first 100,000 cases in the Acute Decompensated Heart Failure National Registry (ADHERE). Am Heart J 2005;149:209–16.

28. Fonarow GC, Abraham WT, Albert NM, et al. Influence of a performance-improvement initiative on quality of care for patients hospitalized with heart failure: results of the Organized Program To Initiate Lifesaving Treatment In Hospitalized Patients with Heart Failure (OPTIMIZE-HF). Arch Intern Med 2007;167:1493–502.

29. Cleland JG, Swedberg K, Follath F, et al. The Euro-Heart failure survey programme—a survey on the quality of care among patients with heart failure in Europe. Part 1: patient characteristics and diagnosis. Eur Heart J 2003;24:442–63.

30. Publication Committee for the VMAC investigators. Intravenous nesiritide versus nitroglycerin for treatment of decompensated congestive heart failure. JAMA 2002;287:1531–40.

31. Moraes DL, Colucci WS, Givertz MM. Secondary pulmonary hypertension in chronic heart failure. The role of the endothelium in pathophysiology and management. Circulation 2000;102:1718–23.

32. Mahdyoon H, Klein R, Eyler W, et al. Radiographic pulmonary congestion in end-stage congestive heart failure. Am J Cardiol 1989;63:625–7.

33. Stevenson LW, Perloff JK. The limited reliability of physical signs for estimating hemodynamics in chronic heart failure. JAMA 1989;261:884–8.

34. Konstam MA, Gheorghiade M, Burnett JC Jr, et al. Effects of oral tolvaptan in patients hospitalized for heart failure: the EVEREST clinical status trials. JAMA 2007;297:1332–43.

35. Friedman MM. Older adults' symptoms and their duration before hospitalization for heart failure. Heart Lung 1997;26:169–76.

36. Yamokoski LM, Haas GJ, Gans B, et al. Optivol fluid status monitoring with an implantable cardiac device: a heart failure management system. Expert Rev Med Devices 2007;4:775–80.

37. Yu CM, Wang L, Chau E, et al. Intrathoracic impedance monitoring in patients with heart failure. Correlation with fluid status and feasibility of early warning preceding hospitalization. Circulation 2005;112:841–8.

38. The ESCAPE Investigators and ESCAPE Study Coordinators. Evaluation study of congestive heart failure and pulmonary artery catheterization: the ESCAPE trial. JAMA 2005;294:1625–33.

39. Jugdutt BI, Butler C. Ventricular unloading, tissue angiotensin II, matrix modulation, and function during left ventricular assist device support. J Am Coll Cardiol 2007;49:1175–7.

40. Cody RJ, Haas GJ, Binkley PF, et al. Plasma endothelin correlates with the extent of pulmonary hypertension in patients with chronic congestive heart failure. Circulation 1993;87:504–9.

41. Rosario LB, Stevenson LW, Solomon SD, et al. The mechanism of decrease in dynamic mitral regurgitation during heart failure treatment: importance of reduction in the regurgitant orifice size. J Am Coll Cardiol 1998;32:1819–24.

42. La Vecchia L, Mezzena G, Ometto R, et al. Detectable serum troponin I in patients with heart failure of non-myocardial ischemic origin. Am J Cardiol 1997;80:88–90.

43. Metra M, Dei Cas L, Bristow MR. The pathophysiology of acute heart failure—it is a lot about fluid accumulation. Am Heart J 2008;155:1–5.

44. Chin KM, Rubin LJ. Pulmonary arterial hypertension. J Am Coll Cardiol 2008;51:1527–38.

45. Ghio S, Gavazzi A, Campana C, et al. Independent and additive prognostic value of right ventricular systolic function and pulmonary artery pressure in patients with chronic heart failure. J Am Coll Cardiol 2001;37:183–8.

46. Di Salvo TG, Mathier M, Semigran MJ, et al. Preserved right ventricular ejection fraction predicts exercise capacity and survival in advanced heart failure. J Am Coll Cardiol 1995;25:1143–53.

47. Kirklin JK, Naftel DC, Kirklin JW, et al. Pulmonary vascular resistance and the risk of heart transplantation. J Heart Transplant 1988;7:331–6.

48. Costard-Jackle A, Fowler MB. Influence of preoperative pulmonary artery pressure on mortality after heart transplantation: testing of potential reversibility of pulmonary hypertension with nitroprusside is useful in defining a high risk group. J Am Coll Cardiol 1992;19:48–54.

49. Jessup M, Banner N, Brozena S, et al. Optimal pharmacologic and non-pharmacologic management of cardiac transplant candidates: approaches to be considered prior to transplant evaluation: International Society for Heart and Lung Transplantation Guidelines for the Care of Transplant Candidates—2006. J Heart Lung Transplant 2006;25:1003–23.

50. Shlipak MG, Chertow GC, Massie BM. Beware the rising creatinine level. J Card Fail 2003;9:26–8.

51. Hillege HL, Girbes ART, de Kam PJ, et al. Renal function, neurohormonal activation, and survival in patients with chronic heart failure. Circulation 2000;102:203–10.

52. Nohria A, Hasselblad V, Stebbins A, et al. Cardiorenal interactions. Insights from the ESCAPE trial. J Am Coll Cardiol 2008;51:1268–74.

53. Henry JP, Gauer OH, Sieker HO. The effect of moderate changes in blood volume on left and right atrial pressures. Circ Res 1956;4:91–4.

54. Zucker IH, Gorman AJ, Cornish KG, et al. Impaired atrial receptor modulation or renal nerve activity in dogs with chronic volume overload. Cardiovasc Res 1985;19:411–8.

55. Mullens W, Abraham Z, Skouri HN, et al. Elevated intra-abdominal pressure in acute decompensated heart failure. A potential contributor to worsening renal function? J Am Coll Cardiol 2008;51:300–6.

56. Unverferth DV, Magorien RD, Moeschberger ML, et al. Factors influencing the one-year mortality of dilated cardiomyopathy. Am J Cardiol 1984;54:147–52.

57. Franciosa JA, Wilen M, Ziesche S, et al. Survival in men with severe chronic left ventricular failure due to either coronary heart disease or idiopathic dilated cardiomyopathy. Am J Cardiol 1983;51:831–6.

58. Lietz K, Miller LW. Improved survival of patients with end-stage heart failure listed for heart transplantation. Analysis of the organ procurement and transplantation network/U.S. United Network of Organ Sharing data, 1990 to 2005. J Am Coll Cardiol 2007;50:1282–90.

59. Fonarow GC, Stevenson LW, Steimle AE, et al. Persistently high left ventricular filling pressures predict mortality despite angiotensin converting enzyme inhibition in advanced heart failure. Circulation 1994;90:I-488.

60. Abraham WT, Lowes BD, Ferguson DA, et al. Systemic hemodynamic, neurohormonal, and renal effects of a steady-state infusion of human brain natriuretic peptide in patients with hemodynamically decompensated heart failure. J Card Fail 1998;4:37–44.

61. Le Jemtel TH, Alt EU. Hemodynamic goals are outdated. Circulation 2006;113:1027–33.

62. Bourge RC, Abraham WT, Adamson PB, et al. Randomized controlled trial of an implantable continuous hemodynamic monitor in patients with advanced heart failure. The COMPASS-HF study. J Am Coll Cardiol 2008;51:1073–9.

63. Magalski A, Adamson P, Abraham WT, et al. Does lowering filling pressures by using continuously measured intracardiac pressures result in reduced risk of heart failure event? J Am Coll Cardiol 2008;51(Suppl A):A80.

64. Leier CV, Chatterjee K. The physical examination in heart failure—part I. CHF 2007;13:41–7.

65. Drazner MH, Rame JE, Stevenson LW, et al. Prognostic importance of elevated jugular venous pressure and a third heart sound in patients with heart failure. N Engl J Med 2001;345:574–81.

66. Drazner MH, Hamilton MA, Fonarow G, et al. Relationship between right and left sided filling pressures in 1000 patients with advanced heart failure. J Heart Lung Transplant 1999;18:1126–32.

67. Lucus C, Johnson W, Hamilton MA, et al. Freedom from congestion predicts good survival despite previous class IV symptoms of heart failure. Am Heart J 2000;140:840–7.

68. Daniels LB, Maisel AS. Natriuretic peptides. J Am Coll Cardiol 2007;50:2357–68.

69. Doust JA, Pietrzak E, Dobson A, et al. How well does B-type natriuretic peptide predict death and cardiac events in patients with heart failure: systematic review. BMJ 2005;330:625.

70. Logeart D, Thabut G, Jourdain P, et al. Predischarge B-type natriuretic peptide assay for identifying patients at high risk for readmission after decompensated heart failure. J Am Coll Cardiol 2004;43:635–41.

71. Jourdain P, Jondeau G, Funck F, et al. Plasma brain natriuretic peptide-guided therapy to improve outcome in heart failure. The STARS-BNP multicenter study. J AM Coll Cardiol 2007;49:1733–9.

72. Valle R, Aspromonte N, Giovinazzo P, et al. B-type natriuretic peptide–guided treatment for predicting

outcome in patients hospitalized in sub-intensive care unit with acute heart failure. J Card Fail 2008; 14:219–24.

73. Kirkpatrick JN, Vannan MA, Narula J, et al. Echocardiography in heart failure. J Am Coll Cardiol 2007; 50:381–96.

74. Rohde LE, Palombini DV, Polanczyk CA, et al. A hemodynamically oriented echocardiography-based strategy in the treatment of congestive heart failure. J Card Fail 2007;13:618–25.

75. Ristow B, Ali S, Ren X, et al. Elevated pulmonary artery pressure by Doppler echocardiography predicts hospitalization for heart failure and mortality in ambulatory stable coronary artery disease. The Heart and Soul study. J Am Coll Cardiol 2007;49:43–9.

76. Birks EJ, Tansley PD, Hardy J, et al. Left ventricular assist device and drug therapy for the reversal of heart failure. N Engl J Med 2006;355:1873–84.

77. Rose EA, Gelijns AC, Moskowitz AJ, et al. Long-term mechanical left ventricular assistance for end-stage heart failure. N Engl J Med 2001;345: 1435–43.

78. Ritzema J, Melton IC, Richards M, et al. Direct left atrial pressure monitoring in ambulatory heart failure patients. Initial experience with a new permanent implantable device. Circulation 2007;116:e1–8.

79. Verdejo HE, Castro PF, Concepcion R, et al. Comparison of a radiofrequency-based wireless pressure sensor to Swan-Ganz catheter and echocardiography for ambulatory assessment of pulmonary artery pressure in heart failure. J Am Coll Cardiol 2007;50:2375–82.

80. Myers J, Gujja P, Neelagaru S, et al. Cardiac output and cardiopulmonary responses to exercise in heart failure: application of a new bio-reactance device. J Card Fail 2007;13:629–36.

Role of the Pulmonary Artery Catheter in Diagnosis and Management of Heart Failure

Rami Kahwash, MD[a],*, Carl V. Leier, MD[a], Leslie Miller, MD[b,c]

KEYWORDS

- Decompensated heart failure
- Pulmonary artery catheter • Swan-Ganz catheter
- Congestive heart failure • Management of heart failure

Almost 4 decades have passed since the introduction of the balloon-tipped, flow-directed pulmonary artery catheter (PAC) by Swan and colleagues.[1] This technical achievement transformed the pulmonary artery catheter from a laboratory device into a practical bedside tool capable of providing continuous central hemodynamic monitoring. The PAC, once defined as "the cornerstone of the intensive care units" and regarded as an important management tool, has faced noteworthy scrutiny in the past 2 decades. Starting in the late 1980s, several reports raised concern about the actual impact of pulmonary artery catheter use on improving clinical outcomes.[2–4] Concerns intensified after a large retrospective observational trial suggested possible harm associated with the use of PAC.[5,6] Several prospective studies were then performed to evaluate the outcomes of PAC use in a variety of acute medical and surgical conditions,[7–12] including decompensated chronic heart failure.[13] Despite differences in study designs and heterogeneities of studied populations, results from these randomized clinical trials have consistently shown lack of any measurable outcomes benefit from the routine use of PACs in critically ill patients. Consequently, PACs in clinical practice have undergone a steep decline in use. Between 1993 and 2004, PAC use has decreased by up to 65% for all medical admissions in many institutions, with the sharpest decline seen in the management of acute myocardial infarction (81%), acute respiratory failure (76%), and septicemia (54%) (**Fig. 1**).[14]

This article addresses the role of PACs in the diagnosis and management of heart failure, the Evaluation Study of Congestive Heart Failure and Pulmonary Artery Catheterization Effectiveness (ESCAPE) trial and registry, the impact of ESCAPE and related studies on the practical management of heart failure, and the general indications for PAC application in current clinical practice.

TECHNICAL EVOLUTION OF THE PULMONARY ARTERY CATHETER

The PAC is an interesting tool that enjoyed an exciting journey from the time it was discovered up to current times. By act of an inadvertent exploration, Forssmann was first to establish the concept of right heart catheterization in 1929.[15] With the intent to deliver drugs directly into the heart, Forssmann advanced a ureteral catheter into his own heart by accessing an "elbow vein" (likely antecubital), and confirmed the presence of the catheter's tip in his right atrium with an

a Davis Heart/Lung Research Institute, Columbus, OH, USA
b Washington Hospital Center, Washington DC, USA
c Georgetown University Hospital, Washington DC, USA
* Corresponding author. Department of Cardiovascular Medicine, The Ohio State University, Davis Heart/Lung Research Institute, 473 W. 12th Avenue, Columbus, Ohio 43210, USA.
E-mail address: rami.kahwash@osumc.edu (R. Kahwash).

Heart Failure Clin 5 (2009) 241–248
doi:10.1016/j.hfc.2008.12.002

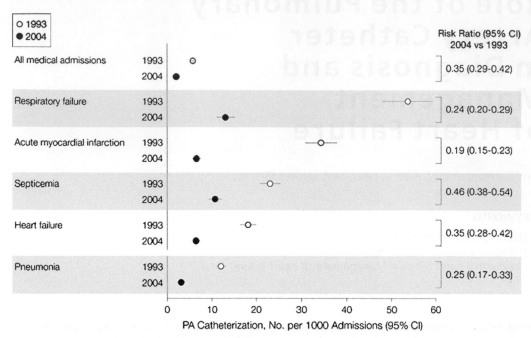

Fig. 1. Trend in pulmonary artery catheter use between 1993 and 2004 according to pre-identified diagnoses. PA, pulmonary artery; CI, confidence intervals. (*From* Wiener RS, Welch HG Trends in the use of the pulmonary artery catheter in the United States, 1993–2004. JAMA 2007;298:423–9; with permission.)

x-ray image; this event is regarded by many as the birth of cardiovascular catheterization.

About a decade later, Cournand and Richards[16–18] expanded the use of the right heart catheter to measure right heart pressures and cardiac output. Their work also provided a better understanding of cardiopulmonary hemodynamics and gas exchange. In 1956, Forssmann, Cournand, and Richards received the Nobel Prize in Medicine for their work in the development of the PAC. Although measurement of pulmonary capillary wedge pressure was first described in 1949 by Hellems and colleagues,[19] the link between the pulmonary wedge pressure and the left atrial pressure, however, was established in 1954 by Connolly and colleagues.[20]

After its introduction in the mid 1940s, the PAC remained investigational and confined to the catheterization laboratories for research purposes and limited clinical diagnoses. Over the following years, two major challenges remained to be solved for the PAC: first, the ability to obtain continuous recordings of human central hemodynamics; and second, transferring the use of the PAC from the research and diagnostic laboratories to the patient's bedside. In 1970, both challenges were achieved by H.J.C. Swan and colleagues,[1] who added a balloon to the catheter tip of the standard PAC, allowing blood flow–directed movement and positioning. This novel idea has indeed shaped the

future of this device. Balloon-tipped PACs not only provided clinicians with the ease and safety of bedside placement via floatation of the catheter tip upstream, it enabled them to measure right atrial pressure and PA pressure continuously and pulmonary capillary wedge pressure intermittently via inflation and deflation of the balloon. About a year later, W. Ganz and colleagues[21] added a thermistor to the tip of the catheter allowing direct measurement of cardiac output by thermodilution technique (using temperature as the indicator). For their renowned contribution to the advancement of this clinical tool, medical communities worldwide began to refer to the PAC as the "Swan-Ganz catheter."

CLINICAL TRIALS THAT SHAPED THE HISTORY OF THE PULMONARY ARTERY CATHETER

When Swan and Ganz launched their balloon-tipped, flow-directed PAC in 1970, the use of PACs expanded considerably and gained in popularity. Physicians now had a means to perform continuous monitoring of central hemodynamics (eg, pulmonary artery pressure, pulmonary wedge pressure, and cardiac output). PAC use was initially directed at the care of patients with acute myocardial infarction, shock, or heart failure, and later extended to surgical units, despite the lack of any solid scientific evidence to support its widespread clinical application. In 1976, the Medical Device Amendments were added to the Food, Drug, and Cosmetic Act of 1938, establishing the branch for Devices and Radiological Health of the Food and Drug Administration (FDA); the intent was to evaluate and regulate the application of medical devices in clinical practice. However, because of some exceptions in rulings, the PAC escaped intense investigation and scrutiny early in its development and its use then proceeded without strict regulation.

In the mid 1970s, reports by Forrester and colleagues[22,23] supported the regular application of PACs in patients with myocardial infarction complicated by hemodynamic instability. Their conclusions were complemented by Rao and colleagues[24] who retrospectively investigated the impact of PACs on reducing perioperative mortality between 1973 and 1976 and prospectively between 1977 and 1982; they found a significant decrease in the rate of perioperative myocardial infarction, from 7.7% to 1.9% ($P < .005$) in patients who required PACs to guide therapy. Additional favorable reports followed and contributed to the surge in the popularity of this device over the ensuing 20 years.[25,26]

The golden era for PACs, however, was disrupted by the first large negative study published in 1987 by Gore and colleagues.[5] Although the study was a retrospective look, the results indicated that PAC use may be associated with an increased mortality in patients hospitalized for acute myocardial infarction complicated by congestive heart failure (CHF), hypotension, and/or cardiogenic shock. In their retrospective investigation of 3263 patients, hospital mortality was 44.8% in heart failure patients selected to be managed with a PAC compared with 25.3% in those who did not receive a PAC ($P < .001$). Among hypotensive patients, PAC use was associated with a 48.3% mortality compared with 32.2% in the non-PAC hypotensive group ($P < .001$). Shock patients did poorly in both groups with mortality of 74.4% in the PAC group and 79.1% in the non-PAC group (not different statistically). PAC use was also associated with a longer duration of hospitalization. Among survivors at hospital discharge, 5-year mortality was the same in both groups. This study has been heavily criticized for its retrospective chart review, case control design, and lack of risk adjustment. Furthermore, it is hard to identify one intervention (PAC use) as causal in such high-risk patients. The accompanying editorial by Robin,[6] encouraged more rigorous investigation in the use of PACs in clinical practice. At that point in time, 20% to 43% of all patients admitted to critical care units underwent placement of PACs during their stay.[5,27]

Within a decade, prospective studies regarding PAC use started to unfold. Connors and colleagues[7] prospectively studied the relationship between PACs and outcomes (mortality and length of stay) and cost of care in critically ill patients. Results showed that patients managed with PACs within 24 hours of admission had a significantly increased 30-day mortality (odds ratio [OR]: 1.24; 95% confidence interval [CI], 1.03-1.49), higher hospital costs, and longer length of stay. This study and the accompanying editorial by Dalen and Bone,[28] were among those that led the Heart, Lung, and Blood Institute of the National Institutes of Health to call for workshops to further examine the clinical application of PAC use in all areas of clinical medicine. From there, the Evaluation Study of Congestive Heart Failure and Pulmonary Artery catheterization Effectiveness (ESCAPE) Trial[29] was developed and conducted as the first prospective randomized trial designed to assess the benefits of PAC use in managing patients with advanced symptomatic congestive heart failure.

PULMONARY ARTERY CATHETERS IN HEART FAILURE POPULATIONS
Basic Management Concepts in the Pre-Evaluation Study of Congestive Heart Failure and Pulmonary Artery Catheterization Effectiveness Era

Before we discuss ESCAPE, it is important to address some of the approaches to managing decompensated heart failure in the pre-ESCAPE trial era. The concept of "tailored therapy" was developed for patients with decompensated heart failure. With the ultimate goal of relieving the symptoms of congestion and volume overload, tailored therapy is a strategy that involves using PAC-derived hemodynamic data to guide therapy and achieve optimal hemodynamic responses to administered dosing of intravenous agents (eg, nitroprusside, nitroglycerin); thereafter, oral medications were adjusted to match the optimal response. Proponents of this approach have advocated that optimal hemodynamics via PAC-monitored selection of the best drugs (and at the most appropriate doses) would lead to optimal clinical outcomes. Preliminary studies showed that tailored therapy may improve cardiac performance, functional status, and heart failure symptoms and lead to better outcomes in patients with lower filling pressures at discharge.[30–32] The lack of a randomized, parallel non-PAC control arm was a major limitation of these studies.

The Evaluation Study of Congestive Heart Failure and Pulmonary Artery Catheterization Effectiveness Trial and Registry

The ESCAPE trial[13] was the first prospectively randomized, controlled multicenter trial designed to evaluate the use of the PAC in hospitalized patients with advanced heart failure. The study intent was to determine whether the addition of PAC-guided therapy to clinical assessment would further enhance outcomes (reduce mortality and hospitalizations) over therapy guided by clinical assessment alone in patients with advanced symptomatic heart failure. A total of 26 study centers with very experienced heart failure specialists in the United States and Canada participated in this trial between 2000 and 2003. A total of 433 patients were enrolled with goals of relieving clinical congestion and improving symptoms in both treatment groups. Patients were randomly assigned to the clinical assessment group, for which therapeutic decisions were guided by clinical assessment alone or to the pulmonary artery catheter group, for which therapy was guided by clinical assessment in addition to central hemodynamic data provided by the PAC. Entry criteria included severely symptomatic heart failure and overt signs of congestion, for which PAC use was felt to be beneficial for management; however, patients still had to be stable enough so that PAC management would not be absolutely necessary or mandatory. Patients with advanced renal failure and those who required intravenous inotropic agents for clinical stabilization were excluded from the trial. The overall target of therapy in both groups was the resolution of signs and symptoms of clinical congestion, but in the PAC group, a pulmonary artery capillary wedge pressure of 15 mm Hg or less and right atrial pressure of 8 mm Hg or less were also targeted. The primary trial end point was the total number of days alive out of the hospital in the first 6 months after enrollment. Secondary end points included exercise tolerance, quality of life, and echocardiographic measurements.

Both groups experienced improvement in symptoms and signs of congestion, and there was no statistical difference in the primary end point. The number of days alive out of the hospital in the first 6 months between the clinical assessment and the PAC group were 133 days and 135 days respectively, with a hazard ratio of 1.00 (95% CI: 0.82-1.21) (**Fig. 2**). Mortality at 6 months did not statistically differ between the two groups as well (10% versus 9%, respectively, OR: 1.26, 95% CI: 0.78-2.03). Subgroup analyses also

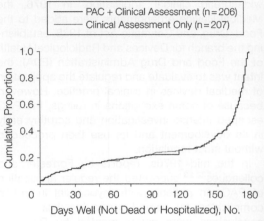

Fig. 2. Cumulative primary end point (days alive and out of hospital) in the ESCAPE trial. Note that the curves overlap for the two treatment groups, pulmonary artery catheter (PAC) plus clinical assessment versus clinical assessment alone. n and NO, number. (*From* Binanay C, Califf RM, Hasselblad V, et al. ESCAPE Investigators and ESCAPE Study Coordinators. Evaluation study of congestive heart failure and pulmonary artery catheterization effectiveness: The ESCAPE Trial. JAMA 2005;294(13):1625–33; with permission.)

generally yielded neutral results when looking at pre-specified factors (**Fig. 3**). Secondary end point analyses revealed a favorable effect on time trade-off for the PAC group, and a trend toward improvement in 6-minute walk during the index hospitalization in the PAC group; however, this trend did not quite reach statistical significance. On the other hand, adverse events were higher in the PAC group (21.9% versus 11.5%, $P = .04$). PAC-related adverse events occurred in nine patients in the PAC group compared with one patient in the clinical assessment group who ended up receiving a PAC later. Most PAC-related adverse events were infection (four patients), with no death linked directly to placement of a PAC.

The ESCAPE trial is a landmark study, being the first large, prospectively randomized, controlled investigation that specifically evaluated the use of PACs in patients with symptomatic, advanced heart failure. As can be readily discerned, the results of the ESCAPE trial do not support the regular use of pulmonary artery catheter in guiding therapy of patients hospitalized with advanced, symptomatic heart failure. The neutral ESCAPE results are in general agreement with prior reports that included heart failure subgroups among their study populations.[7,8]

Several points merit consideration before we finalize conclusions from the ESCAPE trial. First, ESCAPE enrolled patients with symptomatic

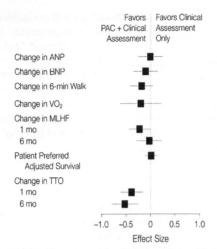

Fig. 3. Changes in secondary end points in the ESCAPE trial. ANP, atrial natriuretic peptide; BNP, brain natriuretic peptide; VO$_2$, peak oxygen consumption; MLHF, Minnesota Living with Heart Failure questionnaire; TTO, time trade-off score. (*From* Binanay C, Califf RM, Hasselblad V, et al. ESCAPE Investigators and ESCAPE Study Coordinators. Evaluation study of congestive heart failure and pulmonary artery catheterization effectiveness: The ESCAPE Trial. JAMA 2005;294: 1625–33; with permission.)

advanced heart failure, for whom clinical management guided by clinical assessment alone was felt reasonably sufficient by experienced heart failure physicians. In other words, patients whose management absolutely required a PAC were actually excluded from the study. Thus, generalization of the ESCAPE trial results to all heart failure patients, regardless of their clinical profile and status should be avoided. Second, the ESCAPE trial did not include patients with cardiogenic shock, or patients being evaluated for mechanical assist devices or urgent heart transplantation. Third, the ESCAPE trial fell short of providing guidelines to choose and guide therapy based on the central hemodynamic data provided by PAC use. The lack of mandated algorithms likely created wide differences among treating physicians in the selection and sequence of therapies (and dosing) for each patient. The effect of this heterogeneous approach on the study outcome is unknown. Finally, the ESCAPE investigators were highly experienced heart failure physicians with outstanding clinical experience and an extraordinary ability to implement their clinical skills in complex patient management. The diminished added benefits of a PAC-guided strategy over therapy guided by their clinical assessment alone may, in part, be the result of a superb performance in the clinical assessment arm (control group). In fact, the rate of PAC-related

complications was lower in higher enrollment centers, suggesting the role and impact of skilled physicians in the ESCAPE outcomes.

Could management with PACs actually alter prognosis or is PAC use simply a marker of patients with a worse prognosis? Recently published data from the ESCAPE registry may be informative.[33] The ESCAPE registry enrolled 439 patients excluded from the ESCAPE trial for not meeting the enrollment criteria, and followed them prospectively. Based on the enrolling physician perception, registry patients were classified into three major categories: "perceived to be too sick," "perceived to be too well," and "unknown." The registry patients, in general, were different in their baseline characteristics compared with the trial patients. Hypotension, advanced renal failure, higher usage of intravenous vasoactive medications, and less use of neurohormonal modification therapies (eg, ACE inhibitors, beta blockers) were more common in registry patients. The use of intravenous inotropic agents was twice as high in the registry patients and considered the hallmark of those perceived to be "too sick" to be enrolled in the trial. Registry patients were considered to be less congested, but more underperfused than the trial patients, as assessed by the enrolling physicians. However, PAC-derived data revealed a similar overall central hemodynamic profile between the trial and registry patients.

In comparison with the trial patients, registry patients had longer hospitalizations (13 versus 6 days, $P < .001$) and a higher 6-month mortality (34% versus 20%, $P < .001$). Interestingly, the outcome of registry patients who were classified as "too well to enroll" was not better than that of other subgroups. In fact, there were no statistical differences between the "too well to enroll" and the "too sick to enroll" subgroups respectively in length of stay (11 days versus 14 days, $P = .07$) and 6-month mortality (39% versus 33%, $P = .43$). This may be because the perception of "too well" was modified by overlooked, important comorbidities.

Analyzing information from the registry database provides us with some insight into the complexity of the ESCAPE trial itself. It is obvious that the ESCAPE trial enrolled patients with lower disease severity and a better prognostic profile than the registry; this fact is confirmed by the considerably higher mortality and longer hospitalizations seen among the registry patients. Another interesting consideration is that the decision of using the PAC itself may have actually singled out patients with high-risk profiles and less favorable outcomes despite similarities in baseline hemodynamics between the trial and the registry patients. Whether PAC use in high-risk patients has an impact on their clinical outcomes now remains to be seen. In short, it is rather inappropriate to apply the results of the ESCAPE trial to higher-risk patients who require more intense approaches and a rather meticulous selection and adjustment of therapies.

Following the report of the ESCAPE trial, a large meta-analysis of 13 trials (including ESCAPE) involving 5051 critically ill patients was published by Shah and colleagues[34] Most patients (52.8%) in this meta-analysis resided in surgical care units. Because of heterogeneities in therapeutic goals and treatment options among these various trials, a random-effects model was used to compare mortality and number of days spent in the hospital among PAC and non-PAC patients. This meta-analysis showed no significant difference in mortality or days hospitalized between the two groups.

A few other trials merit commentary. The PAC-MAN is a randomized trial from the United Kingdom that investigated PAC use in the critical care setting.[8] There were 1041 patients enrolled between 2001 and 2004; 72% of them were felt to require placement of a PAC to guide vasoactive therapy. Hospital mortality, length of stay in the intensive care units, and the overall hospital length of stay were the same in the PAC and non-PAC groups. However, among the study population, only 11% were managed for heart failure symptoms. Analysis of this small heart failure subgroup showed no differences in study end points between PAC and non-PAC management.

A retrospective look at Global Utilization of Streptokinase and Tissue Plasminogen Activator for Occluded Coronary Arteries (GUSTO) II and III trials involving 26,437 patients with acute coronary syndromes was published in 2005.[35] PAC use was associated with a higher 30-day mortality in both unadjusted (OR: 8.7, 95% CI: 7.3-1.2) and adjusted (OR: 6.4, 95% CI: 5.4-7.6) analyses.

INDICATIONS FOR PULMONARY ARTERY CATHETERS IN TREATMENT OF HEART FAILURE

One must conclude from the ESCAPE trial that the PAC is no longer a standard component of the management of decompensated heart failure. The American Heart Association/American College of Cardiology (AHA/ACC) guidelines committee in its update of guidelines for management of chronic heart failure lowered the PAC indication to class II B.[36] The guideline states that PAC use might be reasonable to guide therapy in select patients with refractory end-stage heart failure (level of evidence C).

PAC use, however, should be still considered in the management of acute symptomatic heart failure when conventional treatment fails to improve the clinical condition or when volume status cannot be accurately gleaned from clinical assessment alone. PAC can be helpful when management is complicated by renal failure or persistent hypotension to ensure adequate volume status, organ perfusion, and optimal safe dosing of vasoactive drugs.

PAC can still be a useful diagnostic tool in determining the cardiac versus pulmonic etiologies of dyspnea. PAC data can generally identify cardiac origin of pulmonary edema from noncardiac causes, and distinguish between various types of hemodynamic shock when imaging modalities, laboratory data, history, and clinical examination are insufficient. The PAC provides us with the criteria needed to establish the diagnosis of pulmonary arterial hypertension and in selecting drugs, adjusting doses, and performing periodic assessment in the chronic management of the pulmonary hypertension. Finally, the PAC provides the necessary assessment of pulmonary vascular resistance and reactivity of the pulmonary vascular bed in the consideration for cardiac transplantation and/or placement of mechanical supportive devices.

A TRIBUTE TO THE PULMONARY ARTERY CATHETER

Despite the recent decline in general use, the PAC has contributed substantially to the understanding and advancement of basic cardiovascular pathophysiology and clinical cardiovascular medicine. This simple, inexpensive, easy-to-implant and relatively safe device (in experienced hands) allowed two generations of physicians to directly and serially measure central hemodynamic parameters and study the fundamentals of cardiopulmonary physiology and gas exchange in normal and provoked physiologic states (eg, pre- and postexercise), and pre- and postadministration of various cardiovasoactive drugs. PAC augmented our understanding of the hemodynamic effects of various drugs we currently use to treat a considerable number of cardiac and pulmonic diseases in humans. Categorization of drugs, such as preload-reducing and afterload-reducing agents, vasodilators, and positive or negative inotropic drugs, was largely made possible with hemodynamic data provided by PACs; and our understanding of these concepts and their therapeutic role in human disease helped us develop drugs and characterize their function. We learned from the PAC era that the overall acute hemodynamic responses to vascoactive drugs in heart failure unfortunately do not consistently or directly correspond with their long-term responses and clinical outcomes.[37–40]

Importantly, PACs made us better clinicians by allowing the simultaneous direct bedside assessment of symptoms, physical signs, findings on examination, and the central hemodynamic data and profile.

SUMMARY

The pulmonary artery catheter will likely earn a place in the history of medicine as one of the most useful tools that shaped our understanding and management of various diseases, particularly acute heart failure, decompensated chronic heart failure, and shock conditions. An intense assessment of its general application in nonacute and nonshock decompensated heart failure has now been provided by the ESCAPE trial, a landmark investigation that showed an overall neutral impact of PAC-guided therapy over therapy guided by clinical evaluation and judgment alone. The current guidelines reserve the use of PAC for the management of refractory heart failure and select conditions (eg, pulmonary hypertension, transplant evaluation). In general, the PAC remains a useful instrument in clinical situations when clinical and laboratory assessment alone is insufficient in establishing the diagnosis and pathophysiologic condition, and in guiding effective, safe therapy.

REFERENCES

1. Swan HJ, Ganz W, Forrester J, et al. Catheterization of the heart in man with use of a flow-directed balloon-tipped catheter. N Engl J Med 1970;283(9): 447–51.
2. Robin ED. Monitoring hypoxia. Int J Clin Monit Comput 1985;2(2):107–11.
3. Robin ED. A critical look at critical care. Crit Care Med 1983;11(2):144–8.
4. Robin ED. The cult of the Swan-Ganz catheter. Overuse and abuse of pulmonary flow catheters. Ann Intern Med 1985;103(3):445–9.
5. Gore JM, Goldberg RJ, Spodick DH, et al. A community-wide assessment of the use of pulmonary artery catheters in patients with acute myocardial infarction. Chest 1987;92(4):721–7.
6. Robin ED. Death by pulmonary artery flow-directed catheter. Time for a moratorium? Chest 1987;92(4): 727–31.
7. Connors AF Jr, Speroff T, Dawson NV, et al. The effectiveness of right heart catheterization in the initial care of critically ill patients. SUPPORT investigators. JAMA 1996;276(11):889–97.
8. Harvey S, Harrison DA, Singer M, et al. Assessment of the clinical effectiveness of pulmonary artery catheters in management of patients in intensive care (PAC-Man): a randomised controlled trial. Lancet 2005;366:472–7.
9. Sandham JD, Hull RD, Brant RF, et al. A randomized, controlled trial of the use of pulmonary-artery catheters in high-risk surgical patients. N Engl J Med 2003;348(1):5–14.
10. Isaacson IJ, Lowdon JD, Berry AJ, et al. The value of pulmonary artery and central venous monitoring in patients undergoing abdominal aortic reconstructive surgery: a comparative study of two selected, randomized groups. J Vasc Surg 1990;12(6): 754–60.
11. Joyce WP, Provan JL, Ameli FM, et al. The role of central haemodynamic monitoring in abdominal aortic surgery. A prospective randomised study. Eur J Vasc Surg 1990;4(6):633–6.
12. Bender JS, Smith-Meek MA, Jones CE, et al. Routine pulmonary artery catheterization does not reduce morbidity and mortality of elective vascular surgery: results of a prospective, randomized trial. Ann Surg 1997;226(3):229–36 [discussion 236–7].
13. The ESCAPE Investigators. Evaluation study of congestive heart failure and pulmonary artery catheterization effectiveness: the ESCAPE trial. JAMA 2005;294(13):1625–33.
14. Wiener RS, Welch HG. Trends in the use of the pulmonary artery catheter in the United States, 1993–2004. JAMA 2007;298(4):423–9.
15. Forssmann W. The catheterization of the right side of the heart. Klin Wochenschr 1929;45:2085–7.
16. Cournand A. Catheterization of the right auricle in man. Proc Soc Exp Biol Med 1941;46:462–6.
17. Cournand A, Bloomfield RA. Recording of right pressures in man. Proc Soc Exp Biol Med 1944;55:34–6.
18. Cournand A, Richards DW Jr, Darling RC. Graphic tracings of respiration in study of pulmonary disease. Am Rev Tuberc 1939;40:487–516.
19. Hellems HK, Haynes FW, Dexter L. Pulmonary 'capillary' pressure in man. J Appl Phys 1949;2:24–9.
20. Connolly DC, Kirklin JW, Wood EH, et al. The relationship between pulmonary artery wedge pressure and left atrial pressure in man. Circ Res 1954;2: 434–40.
21. Ganz W, Donoso R, Marcus HS, et al. A new technique for measurement of cardiac output by thermodilution in man. Am J Cardiol 1971;27(4):392–6.
22. Forrester JS, Diamond G, Chatterjee K, et al. Medical therapy of acute myocardial infarction by application of hemodynamic subsets (first of two parts). N Engl J Med 1976;295(24):1356–62.
23. Forrester JS, Diamond G, Chatterjee K, et al. Medical therapy of acute myocardial infarction by application of hemodynamic subsets (second of two parts). N Engl J Med 1976;295(25):1404–13.

24. Rao TL, Jacobs KH, El-Etr AA, et al. Reinfarction following anesthesia in patients with myocardial infarction. Anesthesiology 1983;59(6):499–505.

25. Whittemore AD, Clowes AW, Hechtman HB, et al. Aortic aneurysm repair. Reduced operative mortality associated with maintenance of optimal cardiac performance. Ann Surg 1980;192(3):414–21.

26. Berlauk JF, Abrams JH, Gilmour IJ, et al. Preoperative optimization of cardiovascular hemodynamics improves outcome in peripheral vascular surgery. A prospective, randomized clinical trial. Ann Surg 1991;214(3):289–97.

27. Rowley KM, Clubb KS, Smith GJ, et al. Right-sided infective endocarditis as a consequence of flow-directed pulmonary-artery catheterization. A clinico-pathological study of 55 autopsied patients. N Engl J Med 1984;311(18):1152–6.

28. Dalen JE, Bone RC. Is it time to pull the pulmonary artery catheter? JAMA 1996;276(11):916–8.

29. Shah MR, O'Connor CM, Sopko G, et al. Evaluation study of congestive heart failure and pulmonary artery catheterization effectiveness (ESCAPE): design and rationale. Am Heart J 2001;141(4):528–35.

30. Stevenson LW, Sietsema K, Tillisch JH, et al. Exercise capacity for survivors of cardiac transplantation or sustained medical therapy for stable heart failure. Circulation 1990;81(1):78–85.

31. Stevenson LW, Brunken RC, Belil D, et al. Afterload reduction with vasodilators and diuretics decreases mitral regurgitation during upright exercise in advanced heart failure. J Am Coll Cardiol 1990;15(1):174–80.

32. Steimle AE, Stevenson LW, Chelimsky-Fallick C, et al. Sustained hemodynamic efficacy of therapy tailored to reduce filling pressures in survivors with advanced heart failure. Circulation 1997;96(4):1165–72.

33. Allen LA, Rogers JG, Warnica JW, et al. High mortality without ESCAPE: the registry of heart failure patients receiving pulmonary artery catheters without randomization. J Card Fail 2008;14(8):661–9.

34. Shah MR, Hasselblad V, Stevenson LW, et al. Impact of the pulmonary artery catheter in critically ill patients: meta-anaylsis of randomized clinical trials. JAMA 2005;294(13):1664–70.

35. Cohen MG, Kelly RV, Kong DF, et al. Pulmonary artery catheterization in acute coronary syndromes: insights from the GUSTO IIb and GUSTO III trials. Am J Med 2005;118(5):482–8.

36. Hunt SA, Abraham WT, Chin MH, et al. ACC/AHA 2005 guideline update for the diagnosis and management of chronic heart failure in the adult: a report of the American College of Cardiology/American Heart Association Task Force on practice guidelines (writing committee to update the 2001 guidelines for the evaluation and management of heart failure): developed in collaboration with the American College of Chest Physicians and the International Society for Heart and Lung Transplantation: endorsed by the Heart Rhythm Society. Circulation 2005;112(12):e154–235.

37. Desch CE, Magorien RD, Triffon DW, et al. Development of pharmacodynamic tolerance to prazosin in congestive heart failure. Am J Cardiol 1979;44(6):1178–82.

38. Packer M, Medina N, Yushak M, et al. Hemodynamic patterns of response during long-term captopril therapy for severe chronic heart failure. Circulation 1983;68(4):803–12.

39. Leier CV, Patrick TJ, Hermiller J, et al. Nifedipine in congestive heart failure: effects on resting and exercise hemodynamics and regional blood flow. Am Heart J 1984;108(6):1461–8.

40. Massie BM, Kramer BL, Topic N, et al. Lack of relationship between the short-term hemodynamic effects of captopril and subsequent clinical responses. Circulation 1984;69(6):1135–41.

Using Cardiac Resynchronization Therapy Diagnostics for Monitoring Heart Failure Patients

Philip B. Adamson, MD*

KEYWORDS
- Congestive heart failure • Heart rate variability
- Impedance • Monitoring • Hemodynamic monitoring

Hospitalizations for congestive heart failure are rising and now are the primary or secondary diagnosis for over 3 million inpatient stays per year in the United States.[1] This increasing hospital burden arises mostly because of progressive congestion that fails outpatient management requiring intravenous diuretics or inotropic support to re-establish normal body volume.[2] The cost of hospitalization, however, cannot only be measured in money, but should be considered in the context of how periodic development of volume overload affects overall progression of heart failure.[3] Even though mortality during heart failure hospitalization has improved, with about a 40% decrease in the past 10 years,[4] the overall risk of death is still 5% during hospitalization.[5] Additionally, volume management after hospitalization is a major problem with reaccumulation of excess volume causing readmission of about 25% of patients at 30 days and 50% within 1 year.[2] Therefore, after neurohormonal modulatory therapy is established with beta-blockers and angiotensin intervention, the most problematic long-term clinical challenge in heart failure management remains volume control.[6]

Preventing congestion may benefit heart failure patients not only by reducing the need for hospitalization, but also by checking the progress of disease. Clearly, repeated congestion events increase the likelihood of microinfarction, cause neurohormonal activation, raise myocardial stress, and increase risk of early death.[3] The most successful means so far to prevent congestion is the use of a multidisciplinary heart failure disease management system, which uses physicians and nonphysician providers, and also involves patients in their own disease management.[7] The common theme of heart failure disease management systems is frequent follow-up and contact with the patient to monitor for volume accumulation or nonadherence to medical and dietary therapies. This is important because congestion requiring hospitalization often stems from medical or dietary nonadherence, inadequate follow-up, weak social support, or failure of the patient to seek medical attention when problems arise.[8]

Frequently complicating in-hospital and postdischarge volume management are comorbid diseases and development of the cardiorenal syndrome if overdiuresis occurs.[5] In fact, patients with renal insufficiency and relative hypotension have greater than 21% in-hospital mortality.[9] Therefore, the significant challenges facing providers caring for heart failure patients include maintaining volume to alleviate congestive symptoms without adversely affecting renal function,

The Heart Failure Institute at Oklahoma Heart Hospital, Oklahoma City, OK, USA
* Corresponding author. The Heart Failure Institute at Oklahoma Heart Hospital, Oklahoma Foundation for Cardiovascular Research, 4050 W. Memorial Road, Oklahoma City, OK 73013.
E-mail address: padamson@ocaheart.com

Heart Failure Clin 5 (2009) 249–260
doi:10.1016/j.hfc.2008.11.003
1551-7136/08/$ – see front matter © 2009 Published by Elsevier Inc.

reducing high admission and readmission rates, and developing a means to accurately assess symptom etiology and volume status.

Although organized disease management programs are effective, their inherent limitations relate to the maximum frequency of outpatient visits and the "point-in-time" nature of physical and historical assessments without the ability to examine patients in their own environment. A frequently used strategy for outpatient monitoring includes triaging follow-up by relying on changes in daily weights or development of symptoms to initiate the need for patient-provider encounters. Unfortunately, this strategy is inherently reactive in nature and many times is too late to prevent the need for hospitalization.

Historical information and physical examination findings obtained from face-to-face patient encounters seem effective in delivering therapy, but when these sources of data are objectively evaluated as "clinical tests," the sensitivity and specificity for predicting either cardiac filling pressures or subsequent decompensation and hospitalization are low.[10,11] Daily monitoring of body weights demonstrates significant changes before hospitalization, but the magnitude of weight changes for most patients ranges from 2 to 5 lb,[12] which is difficult to assess in routine home-scale measurements. Furthermore, daily weight changes correlated poorly to filling-pressure changes that occurred before heart failure hospitalization in recent hemodynamic monitoring trials.[13] With these limitations in traditional and available tools to monitor heart failure patients, what would be the ideal monitoring strategy for patients with heart failure?

The characteristics of an ideal monitoring strategy would be continuous or very frequent assessment of the "lesion" being treated in a manner similar to that for diabetes disease management and serum glucose. The information should be remotely available and provide insight into heart failure exacerbations early in their progression so medication changes can be made early enough to avoid hospitalization. The monitoring strategy should provide the means to allow treatment changes remotely or, in the best-case scenario, provide meaningful, understandable information in the patient's hands to guide therapy changes, again similar to the diabetes mellitus disease management strategy of dosing insulin based on serum glucose measurements. It is possible that implantable electronic devices commonly used in the management of patients with heart failure may provide information that meets many of the "ideal" monitoring strategies.

To precisely deliver therapy, cardiac resynchronization therapy (CRT) devices track vast amounts of physiologic information. This information may be useful in monitoring the status of heart failure patients and may provide meaningful insight into physiologic stability of volume status, activity, and cardiac electrophysiology. It is presumed that by frequently monitoring of heart failure patients, physicians can detect problems early enough to take steps to prevent congestion leading to acute decompensation, and thus reduce the morbidity of heart failure. Until recently, however, frequent monitoring required face-to-face encounters in an office, which uses clinic resources and forces patients to travel from their homes. Remote acquisition of device-based diagnostic information is now possible with Internet-based information systems. But what does the information mean and what kinds of clinical decisions can be made remotely, without seeing the patient? This article reviews the nature of device-based diagnostic information, examines how its clinical use can be justified, and makes suggestions for work flow that can make information from implanted devices useful in a clinical setting.

PHYSIOLOGIC INFORMATION FROM IMPLANTED DEVICES

Implantable therapeutic devices, in particular cardiac resynchronization devices with or without an implantable cardioverter defibrillator (ICD), are generally designed to treat important electrophysiologic abnormalities common in heart failure. Such abnormalities include interventricular conduction delay, which is treated with biventricular pacing,[14–16] and lethal arrhythmia termination, which is treated with ICDs.[17,18] By design, implanted devices must sense a tremendous amount of physiologic information to appropriately deliver therapies. It has become obvious that clinically important continuous, remotely acquired monitoring could be possible if the data from these devices could be harnessed in a meaningful and understandable fashion.

Overview of Device-Based Information

Fig. 1 demonstrates the types of information that can be derived from a permanently implanted CRT device. This device typically has three leads with one in the right atrium, one in the right ventricle, and one in the coronary sinus leading to the left ventricular anterolateral region. The atrial lead senses atrial depolarization and provides the basis for the timing of ventricular activation based on user-determined optimal intervals. Therefore, atrial-to-atrial depolarization intervals can be

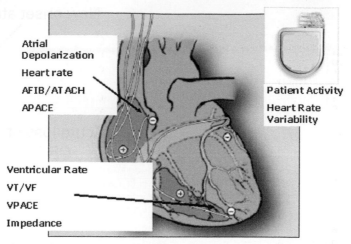

Atrial
Depolarization

Heart rate

AFIB/ATACH

APACE

Patient Activity

Heart Rate
Variability

Ventricular Rate

VT/VF

VPACE

Impedance

Fig. 1. Source of physiologic information as a basis for device-based diagnostics. AFIB/ATACH, atrial fibrillation/atrial tachycardia; APACE, atrial pace; VT/VF, ventricular tachycardia/fibrillation; VPACE, ventricular pacing.

used to monitor for atrial arrhythmias or to calculate heart rate, heart rate variability, and percentage of atrial pacing. The ventricular lead senses for ventricular arrhythmias, such as ventricular tachycardia and fibrillation, as well as the ventricular rate in response to atrial fibrillation. Additionally, the ventricular lead accommodates computation of the percentage of beats that are ventricular paced, which is important to ensure appropriate CRT therapy is being delivered or to make sure right ventricular apical pacing is minimized in the case of an ICD.[19] Memory systems of implanted devices can store the above-mentioned information in addition to providing computation of intrathoracic impedance, thought to be a marker of lung-water volume.

These biologic markers and streams of information are continuously acquired and stored and are accessible to providers through Internet-based management systems for review and for making clinical decisions. By remotely gathering and making efficient use of information from implantable devices, physicians may be able monitor patients from their home, thereby reducing the need for face-to-face clinical encounters while still achieving as good or better clinical outcomes. However, while many device-based diagnostics have been evaluated in clinical studies, no prospective clinical trials has evaluate the hypothesis that acting on device-based physiologic markers with changes in heart failure medications favorably impact outcomes, such as hospitalizations or mortality. Two ongoing trials with similar designs, the Prospective, Randomized Evaluation of Cardiac Compass with OptiVol in the Early Detection of Decompensation Events (PRECEDE-HF) trial and the Diagnostic Outcome

Trial in Heart Failure (DOT-HF) are designed to include several thousand patients to assess if changing medical therapies in response to device-based diagnostics, particularly intrathoracic impedance, decreases the need for hospitalization in patients with chronic heart failure and permanently implanted devices. These trials promise to adequately test the hypothesis that device-based diagnostics can lead to better medical decisions. Audible patient alerts and remote acquisition from Internet-based information systems will be used in the trials to notify health care providers that the OptiVol threshold has been crossed.

Arrhythmia Burden

Most device manufacturers now provide important summary information about atrial and ventricular arrhythmias that affect the stability of heart failure patients. The incidence of atrial high-rate events, such as atrial fibrillation, can discover sustained asymptomatic events and lead to new medical therapies, such as the need for chronic anticoagulation, and assess the success of rate control during activities of daily living. **Fig. 2** shows data from a patient with recent onset of atrial fibrillation associated with rapid ventricular response. The patient was unaware of the rhythm or rate problem. Instead, the patient felt worsening heart failure symptoms in the face of unchanged daily weights or worsening edema. The patient felt his symptoms were not severe enough for him to contact providers. The atrial fibrillation was found on routine surveillance through a routine Internet review. The atrial arrhythmia was treated with rhythm control and the patient improved

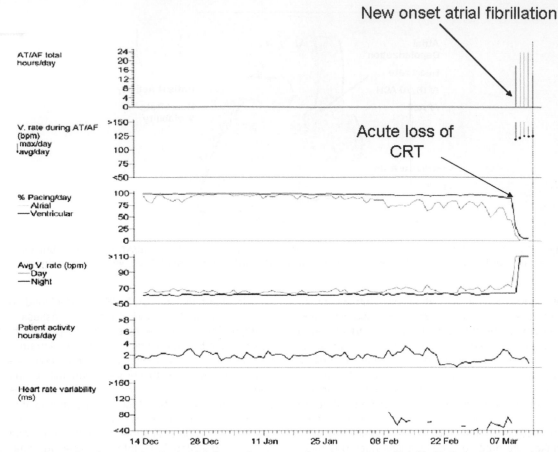

Fig. 2. Example of remotely obtained information concerning new-onset atrial fibrillation with acute loss of ventricular pacing (due to rapid ventricular response). The elderly patient did not sense palpitations, but had acute worsening of his symptoms. The information was observed on routine review of remotely obtained information and the patient was contacted. Rate control improved the patient's overall status. Cardioversion was successful after appropriate anticoagulation. AT/AF, atrial tachycardia/atrial fibrillation; bpm, beats per minute; V, ventricular.

significantly. The report shown in **Fig. 2** is proprietary to Medtronic, Inc. (Minneapolis, Minnesota). Other manufacturers have produced similar reports.

The ability to use device information to diagnose atrial arrhythmias not only allows timely intervention, as illustrated above, but also helps guide other therapies, such as chronic anticoagulation or rate control. Additionally, awareness of atrial arrhythmias may help physicians understand the precipitating factors for heart failure decompensation. For example, **Fig. 3** demonstrates a previously stable patient admitted to the hospital with a heart failure exacerbation. The patient's CRT device continued pacing, which produced a regular rhythm on physical examination and regular pacing on telemetry. Device interrogation helped the physician discover that the patient developed atrial fibrillation at the same time the

heart failure symptoms developed. Rhythm control in that setting was paramount to improving the patient's outcome.

In summary, information stored from the atrial lead in a CRT device can be clinically useful for determining day and night heart rates, atrial arrhythmias, and atrial pacing rates, and for measuring heart rate variability. Information is available remotely through Internet-based information networks supported by most device manufacturers or can be obtained by direct interrogation of the device during face-to-face encounters.

Heart Rate Variability

The ability of a device to measure the atrial-to-atrial depolarization interval from an implanted lead presents an opportunity to measure heart rate variability that primarily arises from the sinoatrial node without

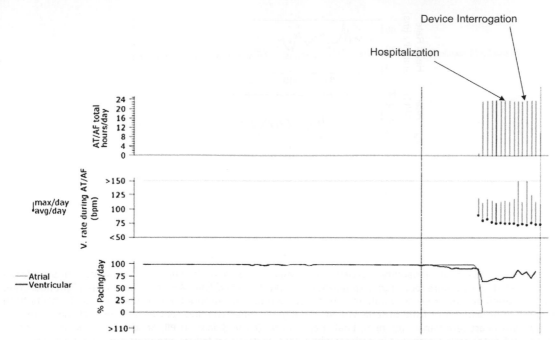

Fig. 3. An example of device-based information obtained in-hospital from an acutely decompensated patient. It was not clinically apparent that the patient developed atrial fibrillation, which was only discovered with device interrogation. AT/AF, atrial tachycardia/atrial fibrillation; bpm, beats per minute; V, ventricular.

the need for complex correction algorithms or noise elimination required for Holter-based measurements. Heart rate variability is a marker of cardiac autonomic control and, in particular, the degree of variability is directly correlated to the "amount" of vagal influence at the sinoatrial node.[20] Higher variability suggests stronger vagal control, while reduced variability suggests vagal withdrawal and an autonomic imbalance favoring the sympathetic nervous system. Heart rate variability is known to predict cardiovascular mortality in patients after myocardial infarction or with heart failure,[21] but until continuous measurements were possible, any association between changes in heart rate variability and worsening heart failure status was not known. Theoretically, it seemed plausible that continuous, device-based heart rate variability measurement would track changes in cardiac autonomic control as patient status changed.

The first clinical study to examine device-based heart rate variability examined the standard deviation of the atrial-to-atrial median (SDAAM) intervals using the medians of 5-minute device recordings.[22] The study involved patients in the Multicenter InSync Randomized Clinical Evaluation ICD Study (known as the Miracle trial), which randomly assigned patients implanted with a CRT device to those with the device turned on for 6 months and those with the device turned off. The study demonstrated that continuously

measured SDAAM was significantly higher after 3 months of CRT in those randomized to the active treatment arm, suggesting that improvement in overall cardiovascular status affected by CRT resulted in a significant change in autonomic control of the heart. This "shift" in autonomic control toward vagal control implies a more stable, less sympathetic dependent system.

Further evaluation of continuously measured device-based heart rate variability included prediction of both mortality and impending decompensation requiring hospitalization (**Fig. 4**).[23] Specifically, this study found that cardiac autonomic control changes to accommodate extra volume as an adaptive reflex as patients progress to congestive exacerbation. Sympathetic activation and vagal withdrawal were identified as early as 21 days before patients presented with worsening symptoms requiring hospitalization. Subsequent investigation discovered that early heart rate variability improvement post–CRT device implantation predicted responders to the therapy.[24] Therefore, device-based heart rate variability powerfully stratifies mortality risk, identifies decline in clinical well-being leading to high hospitalization risk, and predicts response to CRT.

Heart rate variability findings also help advance understanding of heart failure pathophysiology. According to an emerging hypothesis, now supported by multiple trials and different physiologic

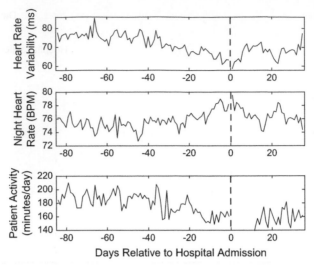

Fig. 4. Average heart rate variability (*top panel*) as measured by SDAAM (see text) in 35 patients with acutely decompensated heart failure requiring hospitalization at day 0 (*dashed line*). Also measured were night heart rate (*middle panel*) and device-sensed patient activity (*bottom panel*). Although night heart rate and activity both changed in anticipation of the hospitalization, the highest sensitivity and specificity to predict the event was found with heart rate variability. bpm, beats per minute. (*From* Adamson PB, Smith AL, Abraham WT, et al. Continuous autonomic assessment in patients with symptomatic heart failure: prognostic value of heart rate variability measured by an implanted cardiac resynchronization device. Circulation 2004;110:2389–94; with permission.)

parameters, volume seems to accumulate slowly over a longer period of time than previously thought. Adaptive changes occur, such as sympathetic activation and vagal withdrawal, presumably to accommodate volume shifts, but the capability of the body to adapt to persistent volume accumulation eventually is overwhelmed and patients develop unstable symptoms requiring hospitalization to return to baseline stability. New information about heart failure pathophysiology was only understood by harnessing device-based physiologic information, such as heart rate variability.

Practical clinical application of device-based heart rate variability

Device-based heart rate variability can serve clinically as a means to assess long-term patient stability and need for follow-up. Data can be obtained either directly in an office setting or remotely through the use of Internet-based information systems. Both the absolute value of SDAAM and its change over time are important markers of clinical stability. In one clinical trial, patients with SDAAM values persistently below 60 ms were at higher risk both for hospitalization and mortality. SDAAM values greater than 100 ms were associated with a very low risk for subsequent hospitalization. However, if SDAAM measurements persistently declined from baseline

values, the risk for decompensated heart failure hospitalization increased.

Limitations

Measurement of heart rate variability by an implanted device requires a predominance of sinus rhythm. Therefore, heart rate variability cannot be measured if an individual experiences atrial rhythm disorders (eg, atrial fibrillation) or if atrial pacing is required for greater than 80% of the 24 hours. Studies generally used some sort of automatic detection algorithm that compared daily heart rate variability with a patient reference line and accumulated differences in an algorithm to detect subtle but persistent changes in the parameter.[22,23] Change-detection algorithms are not always available. This forces the user to visually identify variability changes that persist over time, which decreases the sensitivity of the test in common clinical use.

Conclusions

Heart rate variability, measured either remotely or through direct patient contact, may be useful for stratifying risk for clinical decompensation. Persistent decline or chronically low SDAAM values call for more frequent follow-up to ensure appropriate clinical intervention when needed. Patients with changing or low heart rate variability should be considered to be at high risk for volume overload exacerbation and hospitalization. Continuous measurements of heart rate variability can be a very useful for determining longer-term risk for decompensated heart failure and can be integrated into clinical practice by remote review or direct device interrogation.

Intrathoracic Impedance

Theoretic background

Another device-based physiologic parameter that may help assess volume and clinical stability is intrathoracic impedance. This parameter relates to the resistance of electrical flow through the thorax and is determined by lung conductivity and tissue resistance.[25] Measurement of intrathoracic impedance is possible using an implanted CRT device by evaluating the impedance of a subthreshold electrical impulse generated by the right ventricular lead as that impulse travels toward the implanted pulse generator. Device-based intrathoracic impedance is theoretically superior to transthoracic measurements because the vector and distance between the lead and the pulse generator are constant, which improves reproducibility of the parameter. This makes comparison of daily measurements more meaningful as a marker of lung water.

Intrathoracic impedance measurements as a device-based diagnostic may serve as a marker of lung water based on the hypothesis that pulmonary circulatory engorgement increases as heart failure congestion progresses. Evidence of increases in lung water includes engorgement of the pulmonary vasculature as well as pulmonary edema. Less impedance is found with pulmonary vascular engorgement or pulmonary edema with persistently reduced impedance reflecting persistent pulmonary congestion. In animal studies, intrathoracic impedance declined as pulmonary congestion progressed with a close correlation between impedance and increased left ventricular filling pressure.[25] These findings were confirmed in human studies in which pulmonary capillary wedge pressure and volume of diuresis required to restore optivolemic status correlated well to changes in intrathoracic impedance in patients hospitalized for decompensated heart failure.[26] Changes in intrathoracic impedance were made apparent by using an automated detection algorithm called OptiVol fluid index (Medtronic, Inc.) an average of 18 days before patients presented with symptoms severe enough for hospitalization.

The OptiVol fluid index is designed to daily measure intrathoracic impedance and compare the daily measurement with a 30-day running average, which is thought to reflect the patient's own "baseline" values. Differences in daily impedance values that are persistently below the running average accumulate using a cumulative sum algorithm until an arbitrary threshold is crossed suggesting significant increases in lung-water volume (**Fig. 5**). The threshold of the OptiVol feature can be individually defined, which is important because changing the threshold influences sensitivity and specificity of the diagnostic feature. Clinically, threshold crossings are accessible remotely by Internet-based information systems using data uploaded from the patient's home or by face-to-face encounters using a programmer to directly interrogate the device. Also available, especially for patients traveling outside the United States, is a patient notification system that causes the device to sound an audible alert when the threshold is crossed.

Practical clinical application of intrathoracic impedance

Currently, the clinical characteristics, value, and utility of the OptiVol system are under prospective randomized clinical trial evaluation in two large multicenter trials. The DOT-HF and the PRECEDE-HF trials are designed to test the hypothesis that using device-based diagnostics, with an emphasis on OptiVol, in heart failure management improves important clinical outcomes, such as heart failure hospitalizations. Until results of these trials are available, recommendations for clinical use of the OptiVol diagnostic are based on nonrandomized observational trials.

The first feasibility study performed in 34 heart failure patients by Yu and colleagues[26] found a consistent correlation between filling pressures and degree of volume overload with intrathoracic impedance measurements. In this study, involving 24 hospitalizations in 9 patients, changes in intrathoracic impedance were apparent an average of 18 days before hospitalization, while worsening dyspnea was reported on average 3 days before severe decompensation.[26] An accurate assessment of OptiVol's predictive value was difficult in that trial and is, in general, problematic in trials that are unblinded without objective validation of end points. In a prospective observational trial called the European Observational InSync Sentry Study, the audible device alert system was used to determine if the OptiVol system predicted worsening heart failure.[27] Patients in this trial were instructed to contact study personnel if the device alert sounded and the patients were evaluated for worsening heart failure signs or symptoms. The study found that threshold crossings using the OptiVol feature in patients indicated for CRT therapy was 60% sensitive with a 60% positive

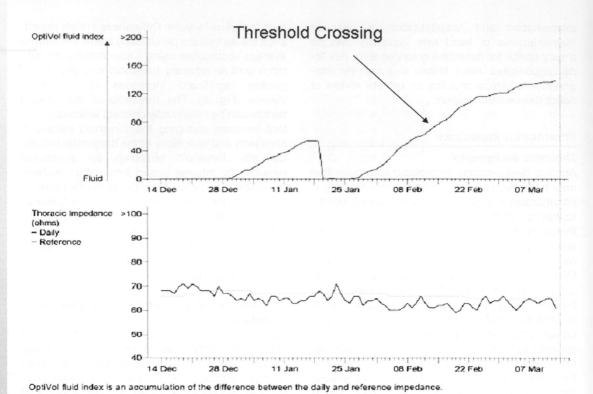

OptiVol fluid index is an accumulation of the difference between the daily and reference impedance.

Fig. 5. Example of the OptiVol algorithm to measure intrathoracic impedance. The threshold (*upper panel, solid line*) is arbitrary and chosen to maximize sensitivity and specificity. See text for details.

predictive value for predicting worsening heart failure. The false-positive rate was 38% during the follow-up period. These results must be viewed cautiously, however, because, individual investigators were allowed to alter the alert threshold or turn off the alarm system, depending on the specific patient's experience. The trial did discover important non–heart failure–related clinical events that cause decreases in intrathoracic impedance resulting in crossing the OptiVol threshold. These important events included pneumonia, left ventricular lead dislocation, and new atrial fibrillation. Other studies also determined that pulse generator pocket edema, pocket inflammation, and trauma each also caused false-positive changes in intrathoracic impedance.

Another small trial designed to evaluate OptiVol's performance in predicting heart failure events included 115 patients followed for 9 months using the patient alert system.[28] Worsening heart failure status requiring alterations in medical therapy was used as the end point to calculate predictive statistics. In the follow-up period, 49 device alerts occurred and only 15 of those were associated with clinically determined worsening heart failure. Interpreting results from this study may be limited by the period of time

following the device alert that patients were examined to determine worsening heart failure and by using traditional tools to determine volume status, which are known to poorly predict actual cardiac filling pressures.[10,11] In this study, the investigators immediately assessed patients to find presence or absence of physical examination findings consistent with volume overload. Immediate clinical patient evaluation at the time of OptiVol threshold crossings will very likely appear normal since the study by Yu and colleagues[26] suggested that threshold crossings may occur an average of 18 days before heart failure status decompensated to the point of producing severe symptoms. Clinical signs and symptoms of heart failure may be a very late phenomenon that is only apparent when patients are well advanced in a congestive decompensation. Device diagnostics, such as OptiVol or heart rate variability, seem to sense changes in status long before patients have symptoms or physical signs develop. This concept provides the basis for the hypothesis that remote clinical decision-making based solely on OptiVol may be appropriate and may lead to less severe alterations in potentially toxic medications, such as diuretics, to maintain normal volume over time. This hypothesis is being tested in large prospective clinical trials (PRECEDE-HF and DOT-HF).

Finally, the first small case-control series of patients studied to determine if intrathoracic impedance predicted the need for heart failure hospitalization enrolled 27 patients followed for 1 year.[29] OptiVol threshold crossing was associated with a 61% true-positive rate when predicting hospitalization for heart failure. Hospitalizations were nine times less likely in those patients with an activated device-based audible alert system. This small, case-controlled study is encouraging, but not powerful enough to adequately assess the effectiveness of OptiVol for averting heart failure hospitalizations. Furthermore, although it may be tempting to alter medical therapy in patients who have an OptiVol threshold crossing without first evaluating the patient, no data are available to adequately assess the safety and efficacy of such an approach. Therefore, until further data is available, clinical use of OptiVol should be adjunctive to direct patient encounters.

Clinical utility and possible limitations of intrathoracic impedance

Limitations of the OptiVol feature may actually provide clinical utility. Other non–heart failure–related acute changes in lung water seem to alter intrathoracic impedance. Such changes include those related to pneumonia, lead dislodgement, pocket edema, and infection. Therefore, what may be a limitation in predicted heart failure–related events may be useful in determining other disease processes that are also important. Current clinical application of the OptiVol feature should be considered as another tool for monitoring heart failure patients and can be used to determine need for unexpected follow-up (when remotely evaluated) or a means to determine early changes in volume that may lead to decompensation.

FUTURE MONITORING SYSTEMS

Devices currently in clinical development directly measure intracardiac filling pressures, which represent the "lesion" of heart failure day-to-day management. A variety of implantable hemodynamic monitoring devices are in clinical trials and include stand-alone devices and those coupled with other, already indicated, therapeutic devices, such as ICDs.[30] Implantable hemodynamic monitors (IHMs) differ in design and include those that continuously measure cardiovascular signals derived from the right ventricular outflow tract (Chronicle IHM and Chronicle ICD, Medtronic, Inc.) and feed data into Internet-based information systems,[30–38] those that monitor left atrial pressure while allowing patient interaction with the implanted monitor through a handheld interrogation device (HeartPod, Savacor/St. Jude Medical, St. Paul, Minnesota),[34,35] and those that intermittently measure intrapulmonary artery pressures using an implanted wireless, batteryless device empowered by interrogation (CardioMems, CardioMEMS, Inc., Atlanta, Georgia).[36,37] These devices offer a new paradigm of device-based monitoring and diagnostics that promise to provide a new basis for heart failure medical management.

Only one prospective randomized clinical trial is available testing the hypothesis that heart failure management based on IHM information is superior to management based on current clinical tools of daily weights, frequent follow-up (including frequent telephone contact by nursing personnel), and history with physical examination.[38] The trial, called Chronicle Offers Management to Patients with Advanced Signs and Symptoms of Heart Failure (COMPASS-HF), enrolled New York Heart Association (NYHA) class III and IV heart failure patients with a prior hospitalization in the 6 months preceding enrollment who were already treated with maximal medical and device therapies. In this trial, investigators implanted the Chronicle IHM (Medtronic, Inc) in 274 patients with randomization to a group in whom the hemodynamic data were used for clinical decision-making and a group in whom the providers were blinded to IHM information. The primary outcome of COMPASS-HF was a composite of heart failure hospitalizations coupled with emergency or urgent care visits requiring intravenous therapies. The 21% relative risk reduction for heart failure events in COMPASS-HF patients managed by hemodynamic guidance did not reach statistical significance, but was reassuring in that IHM-guided management was not harmful and showed promise to be a superior strategy to manage volume in severely symptomatic patients.[38] In addition, however, the COMPASS-HF trial results provided significant insight into heart failure hemodynamic pathophysiology.

Hospitalization for heart failure decompensation in the COMPASS-HF trial was associated with significant increases in intracardiac pressures over a longer period of time than thought probable using the traditional volume assessment tools of history and physical examination.[39] In fact, using an automated detection algorithm similar in design to the OptiVol feature, subtle but persistent pressure changes were identified up to 24 days before hospitalization.[40] Continuous hemodynamic monitoring may provide a superior approach to monitoring heart failure patients in that subtle filling pressure changes can be identified and followed to determine the impact of acute medical intervention. Other device-based diagnostics are currently used as "triggers" to notify providers of changes in clinical status, but do not provide a means to remotely monitor clinical management strategies. In addition, currently available device-based diagnostics are designed to predict changes in filling pressures, while direct hemodynamic monitoring provides a direct evaluation of the "lesion" being treated.

Large prospective multicenter randomized clinical trials are ongoing to determine if implantable hemodynamic monitoring technology is an effective tool to reduce the need for hospitalization and still adequately manage patients with chronic heart failure. The prospective trial Reducing Events in Patients with Chronic Heart Failure trial is evaluating the combination of the Chronicle IHM with a single-chamber ICD in NYHA class II and III patients indicated for ICD implantation.[30] This trial's efficacy end point is a composite of heart failure hospitalizations, emergency department visits, and urgent clinic visits requiring intravenous medical therapy. Approximately 850 patients will be enrolled and randomly assigned to a group in which hemodynamic data are used for management or to a group implanted with the combination device but without hemodynamic information available to providers caring for the patient. The event-driven design with longer follow-up will increase the likelihood that the trial is empowered to make an accurate assessment of the hypothesis.

INFORMATION NETWORKING

Device diagnostics provide a unique opportunity for cross-discipline communication and collaboration. Electrophysiologists are accustomed to examining device data in terms of lead impedance, pacing parameters, arrhythmias, and battery life on routine assessments of implanted devices. On occasion, heart failure specialists possess the equipment and expertise to obtain the valuable heart failure diagnostic information provided by devices designed to treat heart failure. Many times the patient is in a poor communication environment in which the heart failure providers must ask the patient for information about what the electrophysiologist may have said about their device. There are several strategies to ensure information sharing is maximized to achieve the highest quality health care.

Most device manufacturers grant access to Internet-based information systems to nonimplanting electrophysiologists, which allows heart failure practitioners the opportunity to review device diagnostics. Collaboration schemes are unique to each center and require open communication among the disciplines caring for the patient, without a sense of "ownership" of the data. Heart failure practitioners who have device training[41] are well equipped to either implant or at least follow devices routinely. Nonphysician providers many times follow devices in electrophysiology centers and are well equipped to review physiologic data to aid in heart failure patient follow-up. Finally, the implementation of electronic medical records presents the opportunity to simplify information sharing and make it seamless from the patient's home to the Internet then into the single medical record available for all providers.

SUMMARY

Device-based physiologic information and diagnostics have enhanced understanding of heart failure pathophysiology and are remarkably congruent in supporting the concept that multiple aspects of the cardiovascular system change several days to weeks before patients present with worsening heart failure symptoms that require hospitalization to reestablish optimal volume status. Using heart rate variability measurements, vagal withdrawal and sympathetic activation can be detected up to 21 days before hospitalization. Intrathoracic impedance changes to suggest increased lung water an average of 18 days before the patient presents with worsening symptoms. Finally, continuous intracardiac hemodynamic monitoring identifies persistent and significant changes in filling pressures up to 24 days before hospitalization.

These data, when considered together, strongly suggest that events leading to severe volume congestion in patients with chronic heart failure begin long before our current management tools are able to detect changes in clinical status. Early warning of impending heart failure decompensation may provide an effective means to alter medical therapy and avert volume accumulation, thereby reducing severe symptoms leading to hospitalization. Data from device-based diagnostic tools will be effective by either involving the patient in information processing or by remote acquisition of physiologic parameters using Internet-based systems.

REFERENCES

1. Adams KF Jr, Fonarow GC, Emerman CL, et al. Characteristics and outcomes of patients hospitalized for heart failure in the United States: rationale, design, and preliminary observations from the first 100,000 cases in the Acute Decompensated Heart

Failure National Registry (ADHERE). Am Heart J 2005;149:209–16.

2. Fonarow GC, Abraham WT, Albert NM, et al. Factors identified as precipitating hospital admissions for heart failure and clinical outcomes: findings from OPTIMIZE-HF. Arch Intern Med 2008; 168:847–54.

3. Ahmed A, Allman RM, Fonarow GC, et al. Incident heart failure hospitalization and subsequent mortality in chronic heart failure: a propensity-matched study. J Card Fail 2008;14:211–8.

4. Fox KA, Steg PG, Eagle KA, et al. Decline in rates of death and heart failure in acute coronary syndromes, 1999–2006. JAMA 2007;297(17):1892–900.

5. Abraham WT, Fonarow GC, Albert NM, et al. Predictors of in-hospital mortality in patients hospitalized for heart failure: insights from the Organized Program to Initiate Lifesaving Treatment in Hospitalized Patients with Heart Failure (OPTIMIZE-HF). J Am Coll Cardiol 2008;52:347–56.

6. Shah MR, Flavell CM, Weintraub JR, et al. Intensity and focus of heart failure disease management after hospital discharge. Am Heart J 2005;149:715–21.

7. Fonarow GC, Stevenson LW, Walden JA, et al. Impact of a comprehensive heart failure management program on hospital readmission and functional status of patients with advanced heart failure. J Am Coll Cardiol 1997;30:725–32.

8. Vinson JM, Rich MW, Sperry JC, et al. Early readmission of elderly patients with congestive heart failure. J Am Geriatr Soc 1990;38:1290–5.

9. Fonarow GC, Adams KF Jr, Abraham WT, et al. Risk stratification for in-hospital mortality in acutely decompensated heart failure: classification and regression tree analysis. JAMA 2005;293:572–80.

10. Stephenson LW, Perloff JK. The limited reliability of physical signs for estimating hemodynamics in chronic heart failure. JAMA 1989;261:884–8.

11. Capomolla S, Ceresa M, Finna G, et al. Echo-Doppler and clinical evaluations to define hemodynamic profile in patients with chronic heart failure: accuracy and influence on therapeutic management. Eur J Heart Fail 2005;7:624–30.

12. Chaudhry SI, Wang Y, Concato J, et al. Patterns of weight change preceding hospitalization for heart failure. Circulation 2007;116:1549–54.

13. Renlund D, Aaron M, Magalski A, et al. Changes in filling pressures rather than in daily weights predict heart failure events with active heart failure disease management. Circulation 2007;116:II-599.

14. Abraham WT, Fisher WG, Smith AL, et al. Cardiac resynchronization in chronic heart failure. N Engl J Med 2002;346:1845–53.

15. Bristow MR, Saxon LA, Boehmer J, et al. Cardiac-resynchronization therapy with or without an implantable defibrillator in advanced chronic heart failure. N Engl J Med 2004;350:2140–50.

16. Cleland JG, Daubert JC, Erdmann E, et al. The effect of cardiac resynchronization on morbidity and mortality in heart failure. N Engl J Med 2005;352: 1539–49.

17. Moss AJ, Zareba W, Hall WJ, et al. Prophylactic implantation of a defibrillator in patients with myocardial infarction and reduced ejection fraction. N Engl J Med 2002;346:877–83.

18. Bardy GH, Lee KL, Mark DB, et al. Amiodarone or an implantable cardioverter-defibrillator for congestive heart failure. N Engl J Med 2005;352:225–37.

19. Wilkoff BL, Cook JR, Epstein AE, et al. Dual-chamber pacing or ventricular backup pacing in patients with an implantable defibrillator. The Dual Chamber and VVI Implantable Defibrillator (DAVID) Trial. JAMA 2002;288:3115–23.

20. Katona PG, Jih F. Respiratory sinus arrhythmia: noninvasive measure of parasympathetic cardiac control. J Appl Phys 1975;39:801–5.

21. Heart rate variability: standards of measurement, physiological interpretation and clinical use. Task Force of the European Society of Cardiology and the North American Society of Pacing and Electrophysiology. Circulation 1996;93:1043–65.

22. Adamson PB, Kleckner KJ, VanHout WL, et al. Cardiac resynchronization therapy improves heart rate variability in patient with symptomatic heart failure. Circulation 2003;108:266–9.

23. Adamson PB, Smith AL, Abraham WT, et al. Continuous autonomic assessment in patients with symptomatic heart failure: prognostic value of heart rate variability measured by an implanted cardiac resynchronization device. Circulation 2004;110: 2389–94.

24. Fantoni C, Raffa S, Regoli F, et al. Cardiac resynchronization therapy improves heart rate profile and heart rate variability of patients with moderate to severe heart failure. J Am Coll Cardiol 2005;46:1875–82.

25. Wang L, Lahtinen S, Lentz L, et al. Feasibility of using an implantable system to measure thoracic congestion in an ambulatory chronic heart failure canine model. Pacing Clin Electrophysiol 2005;28:404–11.

26. Yu CM, Wang L, Chau E, et al. Intrathoracic impedance monitoring in patients with heart failure: correlation with fluid status and feasibility of early warning preceding hospitalization. Circulation 2005;112:841–8.

27. Vollmann D, Nagele H, Schaurerte P, et al. Clinical utility of intrathoracic impedance monitoring to alert patients with an implanted device of deteriorating chronic heart failure. Eur Heart J 2007;28:1835–40.

28. Ypenburg C, Bax JJ, van der Wall EE, et al. Intrathoracic impedance monitoring to predict decompensated heart failure. Am J Cardiol 2007;99:554–7.

29. Maines M, Catanzariti D, Cemin C, et al. Usefulness of intrathoracic fluids accumulation monitoring with an implantable biventricular defibrillator in reducing hospitalizations in patients with heart failure: a case-

control study. J Interv Card Electrophysiol 2007;19: 201–7.

30. Adamson PB, Conti JB, Smith AL, et al. Reducing events in patients with chronic heart failure (REDUC-Ehf) study design: continuous hemodynamic monitoring with an implantable defibrillator. Clin Cardiol 2007;30:567–75.

31. Adamson PB, Magalski A, Braunschweig F, et al. Ongoing right ventricular hemodynamics in heart failure: clinical value of measurements derived from an implantable monitoring system. J Am Coll Cardiol 2003;41:565–71.

32. Magalski A, Adamson PB, Gadler F, et al. Continuous ambulatory right heart pressure measurements with an implantable hemodynamic monitor: a multicenter, 12-month follow-up study of patients with chronic heart failure. J Card Fail 2002;8: 63–70.

33. Adamson PB, Kjellstrom B, Braunschweig F, et al. Ambulatory hemodynamic monitoring from an implanted device: components of continuous 24-hour pressures that correlate to supine resting conditions and acute right heart catheterization. Congest Heart Fail 2006;12:14–9.

34. Ritzema J, Melton IC, Richards AM, et al. Direct left atrial pressure monitoring in ambulatory heart failure patients: initial experience with a new permanent implantable device. Circulation 2007;116:2952–9.

35. McClean D, Aragon J, Jamali A, et al. Noninvasive calibration of cardiac pressure transducers in patients with heart failure: an aid to implantable hemodynamic monitoring and therapeutic guidance. J Card Fail 2006;12:568–76.

36. Verdejo HE, Castro PF, Concepcion R, et al. Comparison of a radiofrequency-based wireless pressure sensor to Swan-Ganz catheter and echocardiography for ambulatory assessment of pulmonary artery pressure in heart failure. J Am Coll Cardiol 2007;50:2375–82.

37. Castro PF, Concepcion R, Bourge RC, et al. A wireless pressure sensor for monitoring pulmonary artery pressure in advanced heart failure: initial experience. J Heart Lung Transplant 2007;26:85–8.

38. Bourge RC, Abraham WT, Adamson PB, et al. Randomized controlled trial of an implantable continuous hemodynamic monitor in patients with advanced heart failure: The COMPASS-HF study. J Am Coll Cardiol 2008;51:1073–9.

39. Zile M, Bennett TD, St. John Sutton M, et al. Transition from chronic compensated to acute decompensated heart failure: pathophysiologic insights obtained from continuous monitoring of intracardiac pressures. Circulation 2008;118:1433–41.

40. Adamson PB, Bourge RC, Abraham WT, et al. Automated detection of hemodynamic changes to predict heart failure hospitalization. Heart Rhythm 2004 [abstract].

41. Adamson PB, Abraham WT, Love C, et al. The evolving challenge of chronic heart failure management: a call for a new curriculum for training heart failure specialists. J Am Coll Cardiol 2004;44: 1354–7.

Implantable Hemodynamic Monitors

José A. Tallaj, MD[a,b], Ish Singla, MD[a], Robert C. Bourge, MD[a],*

KEYWORDS

- Congestive heart failure • Diastolic heart failure
- BNP • Implantable monitors • Hypervolemia
- Chronicle IHM • CardioMEMS

Heart failure (HF) is a major cause of morbidity and mortality throughout the world, and the incidence of HF is increasing.[1] HF was mentioned on more than 280,000 death certificates in 2005, being the primary cause of death in more than 57,000 deaths in the United States. In addition, HF accounts for more than 1 million hospital admissions each year.[2] The syndrome of HF is characterized most often by symptoms arising from volume overload and congestion, which are the most prominent symptoms leading to hospitalization.[3] Moreover, unresolved congestion often contributes to the high readmission rate in patients who have HF. The identification of congestion depends heavily on the clinical skills and judgment of the clinician and on the individual patient's characteristics. The assessment of the fluid status made by various noninvasive variables such as weight change, jugular venous distension, peripheral edema, and chest radiograph may be unreliable in predicting decompensation of chronic HF.[4-6] Newer biochemical markers such as B-type natriuretic peptide (BNP) help in the recognition of excess volume.[7] Even BNP levels may not predict congestion accurately in some patients,[8] however, especially those who have an increased body mass index, and the use of BNP currently is not practical for patients at home.[9] Right heart catheterization (RHC) is the reference standard method for assessing hemodynamic status, intracardiac filling pressures, cardiac output, and response to therapy in patients who have advanced HF, but it provides only a snapshot of the patient at a given point in time, usually early morning, and usually in patients who have been fasting for the procedure. As learned recently from ambulatory hemodynamic monitoring, hemodynamic changes in patients who have HF are dynamic and often are not reflected adequately by a measurement made at a single point in time (**Fig. 1**). Over the past 15 years, implantable hemodynamics monitors (IHM) have been developed to provide ambulatory hemodynamic data that can be accessed remotely. The data obtained from an IHM assist in the evaluation of congestion in patients who have HF and help in the prognostication and management of these patients. There are several IHM systems under investigation, including the Chronicle IHM (Medtronic, Inc.), HeartPOD (St. Jude Medical), CardioMEMS Heart Sensor (CardioMEMS, Inc.), and RemonCHF (Boston Scientific) devices. The Chronicle IHM currently is the one most studied in clinical applications.

THE CHRONICLE IMPLANTABLE HEMODYNAMIC MONITOR
Historical Perspective

The first implantable hemodynamic device consisted of a pulmonary artery (PA) balloon-tipped catheter connected to a small ambulatory recorder that patients carried with them for up to 48 hours.[10] This catheter, however, was not completely implantable and had to be removed after several hours to days. Development of the Chronicle implantable hemodynamic monitor system began in the early 1990s. Soon thereafter,

[a] University of Alabama at Birmingham, Birmingham, AL, USA
[b] Birmingham VA Medical Center, Birmingham, AL, USA
* Corresponding author. Division of Cardiovascular Disease, Department of Medicine, University of Alabama at Birmingham, 1900 University Blvd., Birmingham, AL 35294.
E-mail address: bbourge@uab.edu (R.C. Bourge).

Heart Failure Clin 5 (2009) 261–270
doi:10.1016/j.hfc.2008.11.005
1551-7136/08/$ – see front matter © 2009 Published by Elsevier Inc.

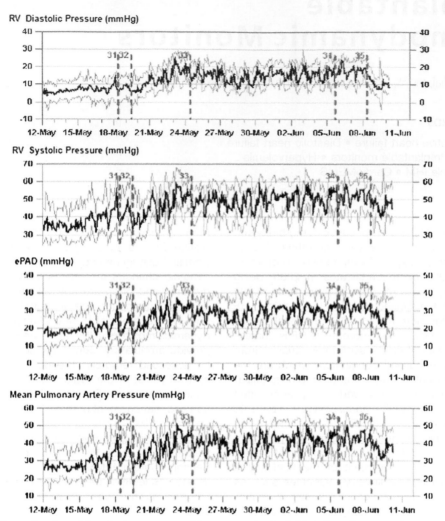

RV Diastolic Pressure (mmHg)

RV Systolic Pressure (mmHg)

ePAD (mmHg)

Mean Pulmonary Artery Pressure (mmHg)

Fig. 1. Data from the Chronicle IHM in a 55-year-old woman who had dilated cardiomyopathy. Note the diurnal and day-to-day variation in the pressures and the effects of volume overload on these same pressures.

a group in the United States and another in Europe reported the initial experience with a completely implantable hemodynamic device.[11,12] The device, which was a precursor for the Chronicle IHM, consisted of a single right ventricular (RV) lead, which had dual sensors for measuring oxygen saturation and RV pressure. These studies were small and had a relatively high incidence of lead dislodgement and other technical problems but demonstrated the feasibility of implanting a hemodynamic monitor. In the first multicenter feasibility study using this implantable device with a dual sensor in 21 patients who had HF, the oxygen sensor failed in more than half of the patients (12/21), but only two of the pressure sensors failed.[13] Given the high failure rate of the oxygen sensor, it was not included as a feature in subsequent Chronicle IHM systems.

The Chronicle Implantable Hemodynamic Monitor

The Chronicle IHM (**Fig. 2**), developed by Medtronic, Inc. (Minneapolis, MN) is implanted subcutaneously, similar to a pacemaker, into the pectoral region. A transvenous lead is placed in the RV outflow tract. This lead carries sensors designed to monitor heart rate, temperature, and RV systolic and diastolic pressures continuously. The change in RV pressure over time (RV dP/dt) also is measured as an index of contractility. The positive dP/dt or maximum rate of pressure is used to estimate the diastolic PA pressure (ePAD) from the RV pressure wave, which corresponds to the opening of the pulmonary valve at the end of isovolumetric contraction when the RV pressure exceeds the PA pressure. The ePAD closely approximates the left

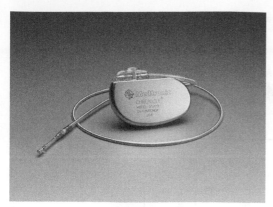

Fig. 2. Chronicle IHM system. (*Courtesy of* Medtronic, Inc., Minneapolis, MN; with permission.)

ventricular end-diastolic pressure in the absence of significant lung pathology or pulmonary arterial hypertension. Pre-ejection and systolic time intervals also can be obtained using the relationship between the RV dP/dt and the R wave of the EKG. The pre-ejection interval equals the time from the R wave to the maximal increase in RV pressure (positive RV dP/dt). The systolic time interval equals the time from the R wave to the maximal decrease in RV pressure (negative RV dP/dt).[14]

The Chronicle IHM contains a lithium–magnesium dioxide power source, integrated circuits, a motion-detection sensor, random access memory for data storage, and a radiofrequency transmission coil sealed into a titanium can. The device can store calculated mean data continuously over a programmable period, record real-time beat-to-beat changes in hemodynamics, and store real-time waveforms when triggered. The Chronicle data are downloaded by telephone to a central computer server via any telephone connection using a patient-used interactive remote monitor that interrogates the Chronicle device via a light-weight wand using radiofrequency transmission.[15] To correct for varying ambient atmospheric pressures, each patient wears a small external pressure reference that calibrates the IHM to changes in barometric pressure. This external device also can be used to trigger the device into a high-resolution recording mode with a reference to the triggered time recorded in the device. The Chronicle IHM data and waveforms are viewed via the Internet through the Chronicle Web site, and patient therapy is directed in accordance with the remotely acquired information. Because most patients who have systolic HF also are at risk for sudden death, the new generation of Chronicle IHM combines a pressure-sensing system for continuous hemodynamic monitoring with implantable cardioverter defibrillator (ICD) therapy designed for protection against sudden death.[16]

Clinical Experience with the Chronicle Implantable Hemodynamic Monitor

In 2002, Magalski and colleagues[17] described the performance of the Chronicle IHM in 32 patients who had HF. The data obtained from the IHM was tested against RHC, under a variety of physiologic perturbations, at 3, 6, and 12 months. There was excellent correlation between the data obtained by the Chronicle IHM and that obtained at the time of the RHC (**Fig. 3**). The correlation coefficients were 0.96 and 0.94 for RV systolic pressure, 0.96 and 0.83 for RV diastolic pressure, and 0.87 and 0.87 for ePAD at implantation and 1 year, respectively. Device- and procedure-related adverse events included one pressure sensor failure at the time of implantation, complete heart block requiring pacemaker implantation in another patient, two prolonged implantations caused by difficulties in lead calibration, one small pneumothorax, one pocket hematoma, and one incision line infection. Showing that the data obtained from the Chronicle IHM were reliable and reproducible, this study provided the framework for subsequent studies assessing the clinical utility of these devices. Subsequently, a multicenter, nonrandomized study prospectively examined the characteristics of continuously measured RV hemodynamic information from an IHM in 32 patients who had HF.[18] The measurements obtained were blinded to the physicians for the first 9 months and then were made available for the duration of the study (up to 17 months of patient follow-up). By using the data obtained by the Chronicle IHM, the hospitalization rate decreased from 1.08 per patient-year in the blind period to 0.47 per patient-year with the use of the hemodynamic data. Interestingly, during 36 volume-overload events, increases in RV systolic pressure occurred 4 ± 2 days before the event. This study was the first to suggest that a clinical benefit could be obtained by adjusting patients' therapy based on the hemodynamic data obtained from an IHM. Subsequently, 148 patients were evaluated for safety and reliability in phase I and II studies in the United States and Europe.[19] This procedure proved to be relatively easy, with very little risk of lead dislodgement (6%) and with a rate of peri-implantation events similar to those observed with the implantation of a single-chamber pacemaker system.

This initial experience paved the way for a prospective, randomized control trial, the Chronicle Offers Management to Patients with

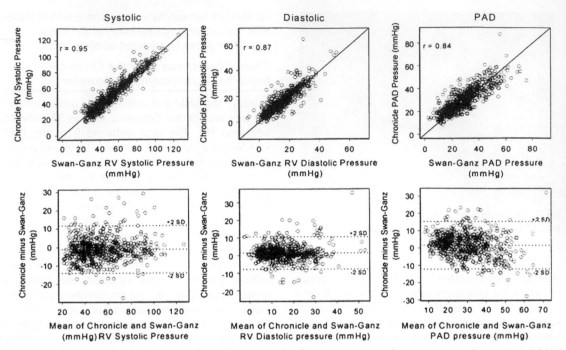

Fig. 3. Excellent correlation between Chronicle IHM and pulmonary artery catheter pressures (*From* Magalski A, Adamson P, Gadler F, et al. Continuous ambulatory right heart pressure measurements with an implantable hemodynamic monitor: a multicenter 12-month follow-up study of patients with chronic heart failure. J Card Fail 2002;8:67; with permission).

Advanced Signs and Symptoms of Heart Failure (COMPASS-HF) study.[20] This study randomly assigned 274 New York Heart Association (NYHA) class III and IV patients who had HF to either Chronicle-based therapy or control for 6 months. All patients received optimal medical therapy, but the hemodynamic information from the monitor was used to guide patient management only in the Chronicle group. Primary end points included freedom from system-related complications, freedom from pressure-sensor failure, and reduction in the rate of HF-related events (hospitalizations and emergency or urgent care visits requiring intravenous therapy). The two safety end points were met with no pressure sensor failures, and system-related complications occurred in only 8% of the 277 patients who underwent attempted implantation (all but four complications were resolved successfully). There was a 21% reduction of all HF-related events in the Chronicle group, but this difference was not statistically significant ($P = .33$) (**Fig. 4**A). A retrospective analysis showed a statistically significant 36% improvement in the time to reduction of the time to first hospitalization for HF in the Chronicle group ($P = .03$) (**Fig. 4**B). It is possible that the study was underpowered to show a significant

difference between groups, because the expected event rate was lower than expected in the control group (0.86 as opposed to the expected 1.2 per 6 patient-months), possibly related to the intensive scrutiny and contact between patients and clinic/research personnel. In addition, as noted in **Table 1**, the effect of Chronicle-guided care was consistent in all but one subgroup, the NYHA classification.[21] There were more events in NYHA class IV patients in the Chronicle group than in the control group. In retrospect, the class IV patients randomly assigned to the Chronicle group were sicker, with significantly higher creatinine levels and lower scores for distance walked in 6 minutes.[22] An ongoing trial, REDUCing Events in Patients with chronic Heart Failure (REDUCEhf), is evaluating the effect of the Chronicle ICD, a dual ICD and IHM, in reducing HF-related events and mortality.

The ability of the Chronicle IHM system to estimate flow, and therefore cardiac output, was evaluated recently in a group of patients who had PA hypertension. Estimated cardiac output was based on RV pressure waveforms, which had excellent correlation to that measured by Fick cardiac output measurements.[23] The intermediate long-term accuracy of these estimates are not yet known.

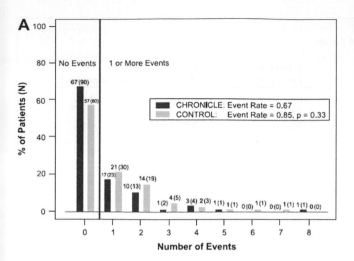

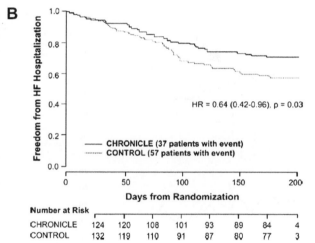

Fig. 4. Results from the COMPASS-HF trial. (*A*) Distribution of all heart failure–related events and (*B*) Kaplan-Meier curves of survival free from a heart failure–related hospitalization.

Clinical Applications and Examples

The Chronicle IHM has become a powerful teaching and investigational tool for the centers familiar with it use. In addition to monitoring pressure and volume status, it has been used to diagnose sleep apnea and exercise intolerance and even to expose those patients who presumably are compliant with the recommended exercise program but for whom the Chronicle IHM activity monitor never changes. In addition, the Chronicle IHM has been used to optimize the settings of biventricular pacemaker[24] to manage volume status in dialysis patients who have left ventricular dysfunction[25] and in patients who have pulmonary arterial hypertension.

The following examples describe a few cases of patient management.

Example # 1

A transplant evaluation was triggered in a 55-year-old woman who had volume overload and renal insufficiency (**Fig. 5**), the patient pictured in **Fig. 1**, with widely fluctuating hemodynamics requiring repeated additional diuretic doses. An RHC performed per protocol as part of the evaluation for transplantation showed adequate hemodynamics (pulmonary capillary wedge pressure, 18–20 mm Hg; PA pressure, 40/18 mm Hg; right atrial pressure 10 mm Hg; all with preserved cardiac output). The patient called back 2 days later, again volume overloaded and short of breath. As noted from a review of the hemodynamic data obtained from the Chronicle IHM, the RHC was done when the patient showed the best hemodynamic profile seen in months (see the solid arrow in **Fig. 5**). This improvement might have resulted in part from her fasting that morning (other than medication) or from better compliance with salt restriction and medications in the day or 2 before the catheterization. As seen, significant deterioration in hemodynamics started hours after the catheterization procedure, requiring hospitalization for parenteral therapy.

Table 1
Results of the COMPASS-HF per prespecified group

Subgroup (% Patients)	Events in Chronicle Group	Events in Control Group	Interaction P-Value (Poisson Negative Binomial)	
Systolic HF (74%)	65	88	0.95	0.95
Diastolic HF (26%)	19	25		
Ischemic (46%)	46	25	0.95	0.86
Non-ischemic (54%)	38	60		
NYHA Class III (85%)	58	99	0.01	0.08
NYHA Class IV (15%)	26	14		
No device used (60%)	37	64	0.15	0.31
Device used (40%)	47	49		

Note that all groups are similar except for NYHA class.

Data from Bourge RC. The Chronicle Offers Management to Patients with Advanced Signs and Symptoms of heart failure (COMPASS-HF) study. Late-breaking trials II. Presented at American College of Cardiology Annual Scientific Sessions. Orlando, (FL), March 8, 2005.

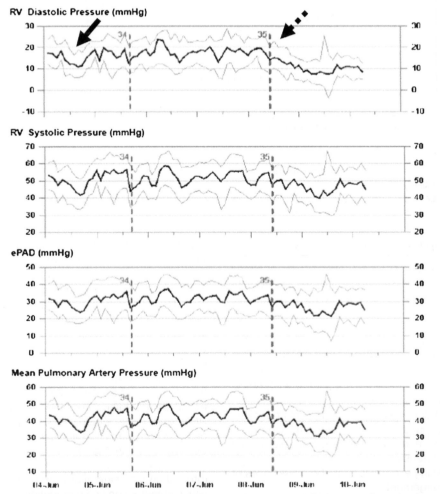

Fig. 5. Chronicle IHM hemodynamic trends from the patient in **Fig. 1**. A right heart catheterization was done as part of a transplant evaluation, with acceptable hemodynamics (*solid arrow*). Days later, however, the patient experienced symptoms of heart failure congestion (*dashed line 34*) that did not respond to oral diuretics and resulted in hospitalization for parenteral diuretics (*dashed line 35* and *dashed arrows*). Note the decrease in pressures within 24 hours of admission.

Example # 2

A 50-year-old woman who had severe diastolic dysfunction from hypertrophic cardiomyopathy underwent an exercise treadmill test (**Fig. 6**). At baseline the Chronicle IHM showed pressures in the optivolemic range. As soon as exercise began, and before stage I of a regular Bruce protocol was completed, the RV systolic pressure had gone from the low mid-40s to almost 100 mm Hg, and the patient became markedly dyspneic and pre-syncopal. These pressures returned to baseline levels within 3 minutes of recovery. This example, again, shows how dynamic intracardiac pressures can be, even in patients who have relatively normal or low pressures at rest.

THE HEARTPOD SYSTEM

The HeartPOD heart failure management system (St. Jude Medical, St Paul, Minnesota) is another IHM system. It is a stand-alone left atrial pressure monitor that consists of a sensor lead implanted in left atrium via a transseptal approach, an external patient advisory module, and an electronic software system.[26] The sensor lead is enclosed in titanium and contains a sensing diaphragm, microstrain gauges, and a integrated circuit that digitally samples left atrial pressure, core body temperature, and intracardiac electrogram wave-forms. The sensor lead is implanted via a superior subclavian vein or inferior femoral vein approach.

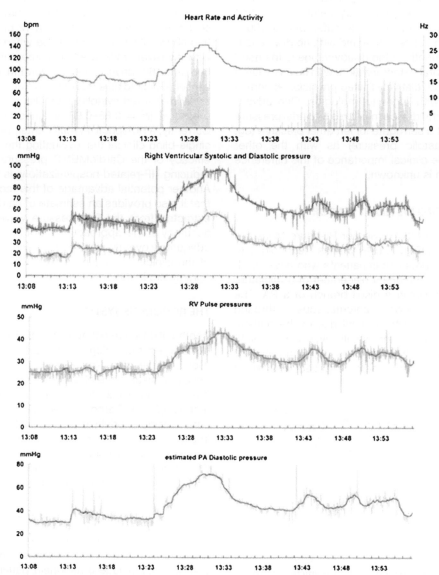

Fig. 6. High-resolution Chronicle IHM tracings obtained in a 50-year-old woman who has severe diastolic dysfunction. With minimal exercise, a significant increase in the overall intracardiac pressure is noted.

Following transseptal catheterization, a folding nitinol anchor affixes the sensor lead to the septum lead. The sensor lead is attached to communication module implanted in subcutaneous pocket similar to that used for a pacemaker generator. The sensor module is interrogated with a modified personal digital assistant called a "patient advisory module." During the first 6 months after implantation patients receive aspirin and clopidogrel to prevent thrombus formation at the implant site. The information obtained from the physiologic waveforms of the patient advisory module is used as input to an individualized treatment algorithm. The clinical feasibility of the HeartPOD system is being evaluated in the Hemodynamically Guided Home Self-Therapy in Severe Heart Failure Patients trial. The preliminary results of the first 40 patients reveal that it is safe, with a 100% implantation success rate and with no device failures at 12 months. One disadvantage is the need for a transeptal catheterization, with its associated risks, and the relatively limited physician expertise compared with other technologies. One advantage is that the device measures left atrial pressure directly, not a surrogate for left atrial pressure (eg, PA end-diastolic pressure) as with the other devices. The clinical importance of this difference in approach is unknown.

THE CARDIOMEMS HEART SENSOR

The CardioMEMS HF Sensor Pressure Measurement System (**Fig. 7**) uses wireless technology to measure PA pressure in patients who have HF. It requires the permanent placement of a miniature pressure sensor in a distal branch of a PA. The procedure is done percutaneously through a femoral vein, with minimal risk to the patient. The HF sensor is very small, oval shaped, with rounded edges. It is composed of ultra-miniaturized electrical components encased in a fused

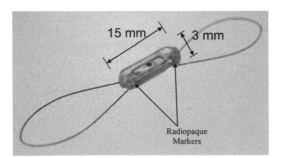

Fig. 7. The CardioMEMS heart sensor. Nitinol anchoring wires extend from the micro-electromechanical system sensor. (*Courtesy of* the Georgia Institute of Technology, Atlanta, GA; with permission.)

silica housing that then is encapsulated in medical-grade silicon. A change in local pressure results in a change in the electrical behavior of the components enclosed inside the housing. The coil allows electromagnetic coupling to the sensor, allowing wireless communication with the sensor without a battery or any other source of energy. Therefore it is possible to measure changes in pressure by interrogating the sensor remotely.[27] Advantages of the CardioMEMS system are the ease and (to date) low risk of insertion and device placement, the compact design, and sensor electronics. A possible disadvantage is the inability of the device, in its current iteration, to store continuous data; therefore data collection is limited to intermittent acquisition.

A recent study evaluated the accuracy of these sensor measurement systems in 12 patients who had NYHA class II to IV disease when compared with invasively measured pressures at implantation and 60 days. The CardioMEMS pressure sensor exhibited an excellent correlation with invasively measured systolic, diastolic, and mean PA pressures ($r^2 = 0.88$–0.96 at times measured).[28] Currently, a prospective, multicenter, randomized, single-blind clinical trial evaluating the safety and efficacy of the CardioMEMS pressure sensor in reducing HF-related hospitalizations is underway. Another potential advantage of this technology is that it also provides an estimate of cardiac output extracted from the PA pressure waveform. The accuracy of this approach has not been validated adequately over time and is not being used as part of the clinical management of the hemodynamic parameters in the ongoing trial.

THE REMONCHF SYSTEM

Another IHM system that uses a similar placement but different technology is the RemonCHF system (Boston Scientific, Natick, Massachusetts). This device measures the absolute pressure in the PA based on invasive, on-demand, acoustic wave technology. The Remon system consists of a pressure-sensing module enclosed in titanium case implanted in the PA via catheter using a percutaneous venous approach and an external system. The pressure-sensing module consists of an ultrasonic energy exchanger, a control chip, a pressure sensor, and a miniature battery. The micro-electromechanical system pressure sensor is used to measure the absolute PA pressure. The miniature battery allows the implant to perform pressure measurements every 10 seconds. The external components include a handheld patient unit and a clinic unit. The implant can be interrogated by the patient pressing the "start examination" button on the implant or by the clinician using clinic unit. The clinic unit also can download PA pressure data recorded on patient's handheld unit. The accuracy of PA pressures has been validated by comparison with simultaneous pressure measurements using Swan-Ganz catheterization.[29] Advantages of the device are the ease of interrogation with an internal or external ultrasonic transducer and (potentially) long device functionality. As a stand-alone system, this IHM suffers from the lack of continuous data storage (as do all but the Chronicle IHM). Clinical trials of this technology and the integration of this sensor with other devices are under development.

SUMMARY

Evaluation and management of volume status in patients who have HF is a challenge for most clinicians. In addition, such an evaluation is possible only during a personal clinician–patient interface. The ability to acquire hemodynamic data continuously with the help of implanted devices with remote monitoring capability can provide early warning of HF decompensation and thus may aid in preventing hospitalizations for HF. The data obtained also may improve the understanding of the disease process. It is important for the HF clinician to become acquainted with this type of technology and learn to interpret and use these data appropriately. With the proper use of the acquired data, morbidity and future events could be avoided with a pre-emptive adjustment of medical therapy, most often with dynamic changes in diuretics and vasodilators. There is a learning curve in managing patients with this type of technology, and mastering the learning curve is of utmost importance in demonstrating the clinical success of this kind of these devices. The monitoring function of the IHM provides data to the clinician. IHM devices, at least in terms of the data-monitoring function, do not treat the patient. Of the IHMs currently under development, the Chronicle IHM is has been best studied and has excellent reliability and long-term accuracy. Multiple ongoing studies are evaluating the safety and the efficacy of this technology in the management of patients who have HF.

One limitation of this technology is the lack of intermediate or long-term data on the accurate measurement of cardiac output (or an index of cardiac output), another important tool in the management of difficult and complicated patients and patients who have PA hypertension. Moreover, acute changes in cardiac output may be missed if the cardiac output is only measured by the arterial–venous oxygen extraction.

REFERENCES

1. Rosamond W, Flegal K, Furie K, et al. Heart disease and stroke statistics—2008 update. Circulation 2008;117:e25–e146.
2. National Center for Health Statistics. Centers for disease control and prevention. Compressed mortality file: underlying cause of death. 1979-2004. Atlanta (GA): Centers for Disease Control and Prevention. Available at: http://wonder.cdc.gov/mortSQL.html. Accessed April 14, 2008.
3. ADHERE—Acute Decompensated Heart Failure National Registry. Q1 2004 National benchmark report. Atlanta (GA): Adair-Greene Healthcare Communications; 2004. p. 1–21.
4. Chakko S, Woska D, Martinez H, et al. Clinical, radiographic,and hemodynamic correlations in chronic congestive heart failure: conflicting results may lead to inappropriate care. Am J Med 1991;90: 353–9.
5. Stevenson LW, Perloff JK. The limited reliability of physical signs for estimating hemodynamics in chronic heart failure. JAMA 1989;261:884–8.
6. Badgett RG, Morrow CD, Raminez G, et al. How well can the chest radiograph diagnose left sided heart failure in adults? J Gen Intern Med 1996;11: 625–34.
7. Maisel AM, Krishaswamy P, Nowak R, et al. Rapid measurement of B-type natriuretic peptide in the emergency diagnosis of heart failure. N Engl J Med 2002;347:161–7.
8. Packer M. Should B-type natriuretic peptide be measured routinely to guide the diagnosis and management of chronic heart failure? Circulation 2003;108:2950–3.
9. Horwich TB, Hamilton MA, Fonarow GC. B-type natriuretic peptide levels in obese patients with advanced heart failure. J Am Coll Cardiol 2006;47:85–90.
10. Gibbs JSR, MacLachlan D, Foc KM. A new system of ambulatory pulmonary artery pressure recording. Br Heart J. 1992;68:230–5.
11. Steinhaus DM, Lemery R, Brenahan DR, et al. Initial experience with an implantable hemodynamic monitor. Circulation 1996;93:745–52.
12. Ohlsson A, Bennett T, Ottenhoff F, et al. Long term recording of cardiac output via an implantable hemodynamic monitoring device. Eur Heart J 1996;17:1902–10.
13. Ohlsson A, Kubo SH, Stainhaus D, et al. Continuous ambulatory monitoring of absolute right ventricular pressure and mixed venous oxygen saturation in patients with heart failure using an implantable hemodynamic monitor: one year multi-center feasibility study. Eur Heart J 2001;22(11):942–54.
14. Pamboukian SV, Smallfield MC, Bourge RC. Implantable hemodynamic monitoring devices in heart failure. Curr Cardiol Rep. 2006;8(3):187–90.

15. Kjellström B, Igel D, Abraham J, et al. Trans-tele-phonic monitoring of continuous haemodynamic measurements in heart failure patients. J Telemed Telecare. 2005;11(5):240–4.

16. Adamson PB, Conti JB, Smith AL, et al. Reducing events in patients with chronic heart failure (REDUCEhf) study design: continuous hemodynamic monitoring with an implantable defibrillator. Clin Cardiol 2007;30(11):567–75.

17. Magalski A, Adamson P, Gadler F, et al. Continuous ambulatory right heart pressure measurements with an implantable hemodynamic monitor: a multicenter 12-month follow-up study of patients with chronic heart failure. J Card Fail 2002;8:63–70.

18. Adamson PB, Magalski A, Braunschweig F, et al. Ongoing right ventricular hemodynamics in heart failure—clinical value of measurements derived from an implantable monitoring system. J Am Coll Cardiol 2003;41:565–71.

19. Stainhaus D, Reynolds DW, Gadler F, et al. Implant experience with an implantable hemody-namic monitor for the management of symptom-atic heart failure. Pacing Clin Electrophysiol 2005; 28:747–53.

20. Bourge RC, Abraham WT, Adamson PB, et al. Randomized controlled trial of an implantable continuous hemodynamic monitor in patients with advanced heart failure. The COMPASS-HF study. J Am Coll Cardiol 2008;51:1073–9.

21. Bourge RC. The Chronicle Offers Management to Patients with Advanced Signs and Symptoms of Heart Failure (COMPASS-HF) study. Late-breaking trials II. Presented at American College of Cardiology Annual Scientific Sessions. Orlando (FL), March 8, 2005.

22. Tallaj JA, Bourge RC, Aaron MF, et al. Continuous hemo-dynamic monitoring in the management of advanced heart failure patients. J Card Fail 2005;11(6):380.

23. Karamanoglu M, McGoon M, Frantz RP, et al. Right ventricular pressure waveform and wave reflection analysis in patients with pulmonary arterial hyperten-sion. Chest 2007;132:37–43.

24. Braunschweig F, Kjellström B, Gadler F, et al. Optimi-zation of cardiac resynchronization therapy by continuous hemodynamic monitoring. J Cardiovasc Electrophysiol 2004;15(1):94–6.

25. Braunschweig F, Kjellström B, Söderhäll M, et al. Dynamic changes in right ventricular pressures during haemodialysis recorded with an implantable hemodynamic monitor. Nephrol Dial Transplant 2006;21(1):176–83.

26. Walton AS, Kum H. The HeartPOD implantable heart failure therapy system. Heart Lung Circ 2005; 14(Suppl 1):S31–3.

27. Castro PF, Concepcion R, Bourge R, et al. A wireless pressure sensor for monitoring pulmonary artery pressure in advanced heart failure: initial experi-ence. J Heart Lung Transplant 2007;26(1):85–8.

28. Verdejo HE, Castro PF, Concepcion R, et al. Comparison of a radiofrequency-based wireless pressure sensor to Swan-Ganz catheter and echo-cardiography for ambulatory assessment of pulmo-nary artery pressure in heart failure. J Am Coll Cardiol 2007;50(25):2375–82.

29. Rozenman Y, Swartz RS, Shah H, et al. Wireless acoustic communication with a miniature pressure sensor in the pulmonary artery for disease surveil-lance and therapy of patients with congestive heart failure. J Am Coll Cardiol 2007;49:784–9.

Hemodynamic Monitoring in Heart Failure: A Nursing Perspective

Erin K. Donaho, RN, BSN[a], Robin J. Trupp, PhD, RN, NP[b],*

KEYWORDS

- Heart failure • Heart failure nursing
- Hemodynamic monitoring • Remote monitoring

As a complex chronic disease syndrome that continues to escalate in both prevalence and incidence, heart failure (HF) creates great societal demands from economic, morbidity, and mortality perspectives. HF is associated with high rates of hospitalization and readmissions. Studies have shown that 30% of patients who have HF are readmitted within 90 days, and 50% are readmitted within 6 months of the index hospitalization.[1] Data from the Acute Decompensated Heart Failure (ADHERE) Registry,[2] the Organized Program to Initiate Lifesaving Treatment in Hospitalized Patients with Heart Failure,[3] and the Euro HF survey[4] have demonstrated consistently that most hospitalizations for HF occur as a result of excess volume and congestion, not low cardiac-output states. Although many patients either fail to recognize or fail to contact their health care providers in response to worsening symptoms,[5] clinicians also are guilty of not recognizing fully and/or reacting appropriately to evidence of congestion. Thus many hospitalizations and rehospitalizations are not avoided.

Even when patients are sickest, as during hospitalization, evidence shows there is incomplete relief of congestion with a significant impact on morbidity and mortality.[6,7] Typically the decision to discharge patients is driven by concerns about the length of stay and the patient's desire to return home, rather than by the relief of congestion and symptoms. Inadequate treatment of excess volume, combined with incomplete evaluation of congestion, has consequences for recidivism, resulting in the "frequent flyer" status of HF that is all too familiar. HF disease management (HFDM) programs have emerged as a successful option for providing high-quality, cost-effective HF care.[8] Importantly, nurses within this paradigm have been shown consistently to play vital roles in improving HF outcomes. This article focuses on the current and future contributions of nurses in monitoring patients and hemodynamics in HF.

BACKGROUND

Managing patients who have HF is challenging and requires the integration of inpatient and outpatient care. Disease management programs (DMPs) initially were developed as population-based initiatives that concentrated on resource-intensive chronic diseases, such as diabetes or HF, to reduce expenditures.[8] Significant improvements in morbidity and mortality were secondary benefits that resulted from these initiatives, and the use of DMPs quickly expanded into other chronic conditions. Even though termed "disease" management, DMPs focus intently on managing patients (not diseases) and use patient-centered outcomes as measures of success. In fact, the American Heart Association (AHA) Expert Panel on Disease

a St. Luke's Episcopal Institute–Texas Heart Institute, Houston, TX, USA
b The Ohio State University, College of Nursing, Columbus, OH, USA
* Corresponding author. The Ohio State University, College of Nursing, 1585 Neil Avenue, Columbus, OH 43210.
E-mail address: rjtrupp@gmail.com (R.J. Trupp).

Heart Failure Clin 5 (2009) 271–278
doi:10.1016/j.hfc.2008.11.006
1551-7136/08/$ – see front matter © 2009 Elsevier Inc. All rights reserved.

Management recommends that disease management should be established primarily to improve the quality of care and patient outcomes.[9]

The most successful DMPs engage in collaborative models of practice using a multidisciplinary approach. Traditional members include physicians, advanced practice nurses (APNs), nurses, pharmacists, dietitians, and social workers, to name a few, who have received specialized training and education about a specific chronic condition.[8] Membership can be extended on a routine or ad hoc basis to other disciplines or individuals. With this multidisciplinary approach, care is coordinated throughout the continuum of illness, throughout all providers of care, and throughout the health care system. Regardless of the team membership, nurses serve as the critical link between the patient, the physician, and the health care system. In particular, the use of APNs affords patients increased access to care, whether it be routine follow-up care, the ability to be seen on an emergent basis, or walk-in appointments. In a systematic review of randomized trials of disease management in HF, Whellan and colleagues[10] found that, although all the 19 studies evaluated were successful in reducing hospitalizations, the reduction may have resulted from increased access to clinicians and increased surveillance of worsening HF that resulted the use of HF DMPs.

MONITORING PATIENTS WHO HAVE HEART FAILURE

Because even small improvements in hemodynamics are associated with significant improvements in HF symptoms, optimizing hemodynamics has long been a target of therapy in HF. Traditionally, pharmaceutical (ie, angiotensin-converting enzyme inhibitors, beta-blockers, and diuretics) and nonpharmaceutical interventions (eg, low-sodium diets) have been used to reduce volume and control symptoms in HF. Recently, implanted cardiac devices, such as cardiac resynchronization therapy (CRT) and a combination CRT-defibrillator, received level 1A recommendations from the American College of Cardiology and the AHA because of their positive effect on morbidity and mortality in this population.[11–14] Additionally, CRT reverses the ventricular dilation and enlargement seen in chronic HF, thus improving cardiac function and structure and the associated hemodynamics. As a result, implanted devices increasingly are being implanted in eligible patients who have HF.

Despite advanced warning signs and symptoms of decompensation, many patients either fail to recognize or fail to react to them. For example, Friedman[15] reported that 90% of patients hospitalized for decompensation experienced dyspnea 3 days before hospitalization. Additionally, 35% reported edema, and 33% had cough 1 week before admission.[16] A survey by Carlson and Riegel[17] reported that most patients had experienced multiple symptoms of worsening HF in the previous year but had poor knowledge of the importance of these signs and symptoms. When patients fail to recognize or acknowledge worsening signs and symptoms, clinicians lose the chance to intervene and potentially to avert hospitalization.

Early recognition and treatment of hemodynamic congestion is crucial to alleviate symptoms, prevent hospitalization, and halt disease progression as well as improve functional capacity and quality of life for patients who have HF. Decompensated patients frequently exhibit a constellation of signs and symptoms, including increased dyspnea and/or fatigue, anorexia, peripheral edema, weight gain, orthopnea, and paroxysmal nocturnal dyspnea. Unfortunately, these signs and symptoms have poor sensitivity and specificity for worsening HF,[18] and their absence does not exclude the presence of elevated pulmonary capillary wedge pressures (ie, hemodynamic congestion).[19] Although daily weight has long been the reference standard for evaluating volume status in HF, body weight also is an insensitive and nonspecific predictor of worsening HF. In an analysis from an implanted hemodynamic monitor that is discussed later in this article, body weight did not increase, as would be expected, before hospitalization for decompensation. Conversely, right ventricular diastolic pressure increased gradually for weeks before hospitalization and peaked around the time of admission.[20] Moreover, data from the ADHERE Registry suggest that 30% of all hospitalized patients who have HF experience only minimal weight loss ($\leq$ 5 lb), and 16% actually gained weight (0–5 lb) as a result of inpatient care.[4] Despite beliefs to the contrary, most patients hospitalized do not present with low blood pressure but rather have normal blood pressures in conjunction with signs and symptoms of congestion.[4]

For these reasons, routine surveillance is an important component of HF care. This approach allows interventions to be initiated earlier, averting the downward spiral frequently seen with volume overload. As the most frequent point of contact, nurses have tremendous opportunities to lead these initiatives, through telemanagement, telemonitoring or remote monitoring, and hemodynamic monitoring of patients who have HF.

Telemanagement

Telemanagement is a low-tech way for nurses to monitor patients who have HF via telephone surveillance and has been used for many years.[21,22] Telemanagement was designed to enhance patient care with the goal of managing changes in clinical signs and symptoms quickly, efficiently, and appropriately. Telephone calls can be made at prespecified intervals (ie, at 1 month and 3 months) for all patients or only for those deemed at risk for hospitalization (ie, following an increase in diuretic dosage or hospital discharge). The most commonly used approach to telemanagement places the major responsibility on the patient, however. Much time is spent educating the patient and family on the symptoms and signs of worsening HF, stressing changes in symptoms or weight, and whom to call should they occur. Because clinicians are not able to examine the patient personally, they are forced to rely on subjective accounts. The result is a reactive, rather than proactive, method for monitoring patients. Not surprisingly, this approach (eg, daily weight monitoring) has done little to reduce hospitalization rates.[23]

Telemonitoring

Telemonitoring, also known as "remote monitoring," uses special devices that transmit information about the patient via telephone or Internet lines.[21,24] The parameters monitored can vary significantly, from weight or blood pressure to data downloaded from implanted cardiac devices, such as pacemakers or defibrillators. Some devices also ask a few questions about HF symptoms, such as shortness of breath or fatigue.

Diagnostic data from implanted devices provide information on arrhythmias, therapies delivered, and device settings, to name a few. Depending on clinical preferences, the diagnostic data may be transmitted directly to the prescribing clinician, to a central monitoring company, or to a third party for interpretation. Recent technological advances may allow the wireless transmission of diagnostic data, so that information is sent automatically and with no effort from the patient.

The basic premise with remote monitoring is that "big brother is watching" or that someone can proactively review and survey data for real or potential problems, and that thereby crises may be averted. The Weight Monitoring in Heart failure (WHARF) trial supported the importance of routine surveillance by studying the impact of an electronic scale and symptom management system on hospitalization in patients who had advanced HF.[23] In WHARF, patients were assigned randomly to a group that received standard care from a cardiologist or to

an intervention group that received daily weight monitoring and symptom evaluation by trained HF nurses in HFDM centers. Although there was no difference in the primary end point of hospitalization rates between groups, a significant 56.2% reduction in mortality (P<.003) was seen in the intervention group.[23] Importantly, this difference in mortality was seen within the first 30 days, further confirming the role and value of nurses in monitoring patients who have HF. In particular, implantable devices and new device features have been developed to improve the detection of worsening HF before symptoms occur, allowing a proactive approach to management.

Measurement of transthoracic impedance via externally placed devices has been available for many years. Because fluid is a good conductor of electricity, increasing volume within the pulmonary circulation results in reduced impedance. The widespread usefulness of transthoracic impedance has been limited by the acquisition of data at a single time-point. Recent advances have made it possible to measure and collect longitudinal data about intrathoracic impedance through an implanted combination CRT-defibrillator.[25] Clinical investigations of this feature have shown that reductions in impedance preceded hospitalization and symptoms of worsening HF by an average of 21 days, serving as an early warning of increasing congestion and the need for prompt intervention to avoid hospitalization.[26,27] The Prospective, Randomized, Evaluation of Cardiac Compass with OptiVol in the Early Detection of Decompensation Events for Heart Failure is an ongoing prospective, randomized, controlled trial designed to evaluate the efficacy of intrathoracic fluid monitoring to reduce hospitalization in patients who have HF. In most practice settings, nurses have taken the lead in using this data, in conjunction with other device diagnostics, to manage their patients proactively.[28]

The Remote Active Monitoring in Patients with Heart Failure trial is designed to evaluate use of wireless technology in making treatment decisions and the impact on patient outcomes such as hospitalizations, HF events, and mortality.[29] This trial uses the Latitude system (Boston-Scientific, St. Paul, MN), which collects information on patient symptoms, weight, blood pressure, activity, heart rate variability, and arrhythmias.

Although telemonitoring may improve morbidity, mortality, or both in patients who have HF,[23,24,30] it is important to acknowledge some of the limitations associated with this approach, including the need for 24-hour availability to receive and interpret transmitted data, patient adherence to telemonitoring instructions and schedules, and any liability associated with time delays between data transmission, treatment decisions, and communication to the patient.

Hemodynamic monitoring

As previously stated, the management of HF historically has been reactive in nature. The ability to monitor ambulatory hemodynamic parameters can be beneficial, because early subclinical congestion can be detected and treated, in some cases before the patient recognizes any symptoms.[6,20] Beyond implantable impedance monitoring, the next generation of implanted devices are likely to include hemodynamic monitoring systems. In addition to providing early warning of worsening HF, these devices may provide a day-to-day management system for patients. Continuous monitoring of patients and therapy tailored to individualized clinical and hemodynamic profiles have been shown to limit the symptoms of HF.[31–33] A number of implantable hemodynamic monitoring (IHM) devices and systems are currently under investigation, but none currently have approval from the Food and Drug Administration (FDA).

These IHM devices allow the continuous or intermittent assessment of hemodynamics, generally focusing on the direct measurement or estimation of left-sided filling pressure. These devices are predicated on observations that there may be a prolonged period of slow deterioration (ie, fluid retention and the development of hemodynamic congestion) that occurs over days to weeks before symptoms and subsequent overt decompensation ensue.[6] Following is information on some of the IHMs currently under clinical investigation.

The Chronicle IHM (Medtronic Inc., Minneapolis, MN) uses a single lead in the right ventricular outflow track to record hemodynamic measurements. The device measures continuous right ventricular systolic and diastolic pressures and provides an estimate of the pulmonary artery diastolic pressure. Data are transmitted to a secure Web site, where clinicians view and use the data for clinical decision making. The Chronicle IHM has been evaluated and validated extensively, demonstrating its accuracy in measuring hemodynamic parameters.[6,34] Data from Chronicle Offers Management of Patients with Advanced Signs and Symptoms of Heart Failure trial, a 274-patient, phase III randomized, controlled trial, support the potential utility of this approach in managing patients who have HF.[30] Monitoring of hemodynamic data is combined with therapy in the Reducing Decompensation Events Using Intracardiac Pressures in Patients with Chronic HF (REDUCEhf) clinical trial.[35] The REDUCEhf trial

is designed to evaluate the efficacy of Chronicle IHM-guided care in reducing HF-related events in patients needing a single-lead defibrillator. In the control group of the REDUCEhf trial, clinicians are blinded to hemodynamic data, and patients receive "standard care" based on symptoms and other usual parameters. In the treatment group, however, clinicians have access to chronic hemodynamic data to optimize volume status and to minimize symptoms. Of importance, the defibrillator will be active in all patients, regardless of group assignment.

A variety of hemodynamic monitors using sensors placed in essentially every chamber of the heart are under investigation. In addition to the right ventricle discussed earlier in this article, sensors are being implanted in the pulmonary artery, left atrium, and left ventricle. Theoretically, in the future clinicians may be able to select a particular chamber to be monitored, based on a patient's underlying disease process. These devices also provide diagnostic, therapeutic, and prognostic information for the treatment of HF.[34,36]

Some of the hemodynamic monitors offer patients some control over their own disease through self-management of hemodynamic data. This control is similar to diabetics' self-management of glucose levels using a glucometer. The Hemodynamically Guided Home Self-Therapy In Severe HF Patients clinical trial (St. Jude Medical, St. Paul, MN), places a dime-size sensor in the left atrium to measure pressures directly.[37] Patients are instructed to check their left atrial pressures twice a day using a special handheld device. This device then provides individualized instructions for managing left atrial pressure and hemodynamic targets, as determined by their clinician. For example, if the left atrial pressure is 20 mm Hg, the patient may be instructed to avoid exertional activities, take a particular dosage of a diuretic, and to recheck the left atrial pressure in 6 hours. The potential for IHM devices to revolutionize the management of HF is substantial but remains under investigation. **Table 1** lists implanted hemodynamic monitors currently under investigation.

NURSING PERSPECTIVES IN THE HEMODYNAMIC MONITORING OF HEART FAILURE

The role of nurses in managing patients with HF is well established, and nurses must accept and adopt technology into their clinical routines and practices. It is important to acknowledge that the benefits seen with implanted devices are additive to medications. Angiotensin-converting enzyme inhibitors and specific beta-blockers constitute the cornerstones of medical therapy, because

Table 1
Implanted hemodynamic monitors undergoing clinical investigation

Device Name (Company and Location)	Components	Sensor Location	Parameters Measured
Chronicle IHM (Medtronic Inc., Minneapolis, MN)	32K monitor memory unit Tined ventricular lead with 02 saturation sensor and pressure transducer External pressure reference recorder External programmer	RV outflow track	Heart rate Right ventricular systolic/diastolic pressure Estimated PA diastolic pressure Right ventricular pulse pressure RV contractility (dP/dt) Physical activity
Savacor HeartPod (St. Jude Medical Inc., Sylmar, CA)	Implantable sensor system External patient advisory monitor Dynamic prescription software	Left atrium	Direct left atrial pressure Core body temperature Intracardiac EKG
HeartSure (CardioMEMS, Atlanta, GA)	Wireless sensor with functional components within sensor capsule External antenna Interrogation system	Pulmonary artery	Heart rate Pulmonary artery systolic/diastolic pressures Cardiac output
Remon (Boston Scientific Inc., St. Paul, MN)	Pressure sensor Piezoelectric transducer Low-power control chip External communication/analysis unit	Pulmonary artery	Pulmonary artery systolic/diastolic pressures

Abbreviations: PA, pulmonary artery; RV, right ventricular.

they provide neurohormonal blockade, halt disease progression, and reduce the morbidity and mortality seen in HF. These life-saving medications should be initiated and titrated to the maximally tolerated doses, using targets of the doses demonstrating efficacy in randomized, controlled clinical trials.[11] Once these medications have been optimized, the indications for implanted devices should be considered. Through the use of disease management models, multidisciplinary care, and increased access to health care providers, nurses are well positioned to continue as the leaders in telemanagement and telemonitoring in HF.

When IHMs, receive FDA approval, managing HF will change dramatically. Because many different IHMs, monitoring a variety of intracardiac chambers and examining a number of primary end points, currently are undergoing clinical investigation, it is likely that one or more devices will receive FDA approval in the near future (see **Table 1**). For this reason, clinicians must understand how the hemodynamic data obtained from patients who have implanted devices differ

significantly from the hemodynamic data obtained in an acute care environment. During hospitalization, information on filling pressures is collected for a short time period in an "artificial" setting, because the patient is primarily bedridden. In contrast, the implanted devices collect data continuously while the patient is engaging in normal daily activities at home.

New technology can be intimidating, however, especially if its use alters routine practices or protocols. Nurses must become familiar with the parameters being measured by implanted devices and their clinical implications. Critical thinking skills for data interpretation and clinical decision making must be developed. Doing so will take some time, and thus networking and learning from those involved with the clinical investigations of devices will be extremely helpful and important. Rigorous monitoring for changes that can occur with sodium indiscretion, arrhythmias, angina, activity, or nonadherence to prescribed therapies will be central to avoid morbidity and mortality. Trusting this new information and learning how to react, especially in the absence of patient symptoms, will be difficult initially. Comfort in using the technology will increase as improved patient outcomes and symptoms result.

In addition to the learning curve required for using new technology, workflow is an important consideration. Processes for the delineation of responsibilities should be established before the implantation of a device with hemodynamic capacities. Adequate resources to support the proactive model, including equipment, personnel, and allocated time, are essential to success. Failure to provide these resources will result in staff frustration, unchanged practice patterns, and inappropriate device selection. Implementing the team approach with HF and electrophysiology (EP) staff will produce efficiencies in the system and better patient outcomes.[38] One simple initial step would be to coordinate follow-up visits, so that patients who have HF monitored by implanted devices can be seen by HF and EP staff on the same day. Enhanced communication about implanted device interrogations, the interpretation of hemodynamic data, and changes in the treatment plan are anticipated results. Savings in time, transportation expenses, and lost income are positive consequences for the patient, family, or both. IHMs may offer additional benefit to patients who have advanced HF and in particular to older patients who find it physically difficult make appointments and do not seek medical assistance in a timely manner.[31]

Finally, although the expenditure of time and resources associated with these devices is significant, reimbursement for remote monitoring is lagging. In addition to HF, a number of other chronic conditions, including sleep disorders, diabetes, and arrhythmias, use remote monitoring. Legislation entitled the "Remote Monitoring Access Act" has been making its way through Congress for the past several years.[39] The most recent version of the legislation, presented on November 6, 2007 (S. 631) is pending and requires national Medicare coverage for HF and cardiac arrhythmias, with implementation delayed until 2009.[40] The Medicare bill is expected to come up for a vote by the end of 2008.

As the most common and frequent point of contact for patients, nurses are well positioned to take a leading role in this change. Educating other health care providers, such as physicians, APNs, physician assistants, and other nurses about IHM devices and about important physiologic parameters and their clinical implications for patients will be a key strategy. A shift from the present reactive to a more proactive model for managing HF will occur only when those involved trust and use the data to individualize HF treatment. Therefore, nurses must not become complacent about HF and must continually learn about contemporary evidence-based HF care, upcoming clinical trials, recently approved drugs or devices, and other technological advances.

SUMMARY

Until evidence from clinical trials of IHMs is available and approval from the FDA is received, the best available model seems to be telemonitoring in conjunction with a comprehensive HFDMP. A number of issues, including established processes for data review and decision-making and reimbursement, must be addressed before telemonitoring and IHM are widely adopted and accepted. Nurses, as the most frequent and common contact for patients, have the ability and opportunity to lead this change.

REFERENCES

1. Cleland JG, Gemmell I, Khand A, et al. Is the prognosis of heart failure improving? Eur J Heart Fail 1999;1:229–41.
2. The Adhere Scientific Advisory Committee. Insights from the Acute Decompensated Heart Failure National Registry (ADHERE REGISTRY): data from 96094 patient cases. Available at: http://www.adhereregistry.com/ADHEREQ102BMR_Final.pdf. Accessed January 3, 2008.
3. Fonarow GC, Abraham WT, Albert NM, et al. Influence of a performance-improvement initiative on quality of care for patients hospitalized with heart failure: results of the organized program to initiate lifesaving treatment in hospitalized patients with heart failure (OPTIMIZE-HF). Arch Intern Med 2007;167:1493–502.
4. Hobbs FD, Jones MI, Wilson S, et al. European survey of primary care physician perceptions on heart failure diagnosis and management (Euro-HF). Eur Heart J 2000;21(22):1877–87.
5. Friedman M, Griffin JA. Relationship of physical symptoms and physical functioning to depression in patients with heart failure. Heart Lung 2001; 30(2):98–104.
6. Adamson PB, Magalski A, Braunschweig F, et al. Ongoing right ventricular hemodynamics in heart failure: clinical value of measurements derived from an implantable monitoring system. J Am Coll Cardiol 2003;41:565–71.
7. Fonarow GC, On behalf of the ADHERE Steering Committee. The Acute Decompensated Heart Failure Registry (ADHERE): opportunities to improve care of patients hospitalized with acute decompensated heart failure. Rev Cardiovasc Med 2003;4:S21–30.

8. Trupp RJ. Disease management overview. In: Abraham WT, Krum H, editors. Heart failure: a practical approach to therapy. Chicago: McGraw-Hill 2007:241–52.

9. Faxon DP, Schwamm LH, Pasternak R, et al. Improving quality of care through disease management: principles and recommendations from the American Heart Association's Expert Panel on Disease Management. Circulation 2003; 109:2651–4.

10. Whellan D, Hasselbad V, Peterson E, et al. Metaanalysis and review of heart failure disease management randomized controlled clinical studies. Am Heart J 2005;149(4):722–9.

11. Hunt SA, Abraham WT, Chin MH, et al. ACC/AHA 2005 guideline update for the diagnosis and management of chronic heart failure in the adult–summary article. Circulation 2005;112:1825–52.

12. Abraham WT, Fisher WG, Smith AL, et al. Cardiac resynchronization in chronic heart failure. N Engl J Med 2002;346:1845–53.

13. Bristow MR, Saxon LA, Boehmer J, et al. Cardiac resynchronization therapy with or without implantable defibrillator in advanced heart failure. N Engl J Med 2004;350:2140–50.

14. Moss AJ, Zareba W, Hall WJ, et al. Prophylactic implantation of a defibrillator in patients with myocardial infarction and reduced ejection fraction. N Engl J Med 2002;346:877–83.

15. Friedman MM. Older adults' symptoms and their duration before hospitalization for heart failure. Heart Lung 1997;26(3):169–76.

16. Vinson J, Rich MW, Sperry JC, et al. Early readmission of elderly patients with congestive heart failure. J Am Geriatr Soc 1990;38:1290–5.

17. Carlson B, Riegel B. Self-care abilities of patients with heart failure. Heart Lung 2001;30(5):351–9.

18. Roccaforte R, Demers C, Baldassarre F, et al. Effectiveness of comprehensive disease management programmes in improving clinical outcomes in heart failure patients. A meta-analysis. Eur J Heart Fail 2005;7:1133–44.

19. Dao Q, Krishnaswamy P, Kazanegra R, et al. Utility of B-type natriuretic peptide in the diagnosis of congestive heart failure in an urgent care setting. J Am Coll Cardiol 2001;37:379–85.

20. Stevenson LW, Perloff JK. The limited reliability of physical signs for estimating hemodynamics in chronic heart failure. JAMA 1989;261:884.

21. Adamson PB, Magalski A, Bourge RC, et al. Relationship between right ventricular pressures variability and heart failure related adverse events. J Am Coll Cardiol 2003;41(6):suppl 1, 58.

22. Clark RA, Inglis SC, McAlister FA, et al. Telemonitoring or structured telephone support programmes for patients with chronic heart failure: systematic review and meta-analysis. 2007. Available at: http://www.bmj.com/cgi/rapidpdf/bmj.39156.536968.55v1. Accessed January 8, 2008.

23. Bondmass M, Bolger N, Castro G, et al. The effect of physiologic home monitoring and telemanagement on chronic heart failure outcomes. 2002. Internet Journal of Advanced Nursing Practice 2002. Available at: http://ispub.com/journals/IJANP/Vol3N2?chf.htm. Accessed January 10, 2008.

24. Goldberg LR, Piette JD, Walsh MN, et al. Randomized trial of a daily electronic home monitoring system in patients with advanced heart failure: the Weight Monitoring in Heart Failure (WHARF) trial. Am Heart J 2003;146:705–12.

25. Louis A, Turner T, Gretton M, et al. A systematic review of telemonitoring for the management of heart failure. The Eur J Heart Fail 2003;5:583–90.

26. Rathman L, Repoley J, Delgado S, et al. Using devices for physiologic monitoring in heart failure. Journal of Cardiovascular Nursing 2008;23(2):159–68.

27. Yu CM, Wang L, Chau E, et al. Intrathoracic impedance monitoring in patients with heart failure. Circulation 2005;112:841–8.

28. Abraham WT, Foreman B, Fishel R, et al. Fluid Accumulation Status Trial (FAST). Heart Rhythm 2005; 2(suppl):S65 [abstract AB33–4].

29. Rathman L, Repoley J, Tubbs K, et al. Monitoring intrathoracic impedance with CRT-D devices: insight into volume status. Prog Cardiovasc Nurs 2006; 21(2):97–9.

30. Saxon LA. Remote active monitoring in patients with heart failure (RAPID-HF): design and rationale. J Card Fail 2007;13(4):241–6.

31. Bourge RC, Abraham WT, Aaron M, et al. Preliminary results of the COMPASS-HF Trial. Presented at a late-breaking clinical trials session at the 78th Annual Scientific Sessions of the American Heart Association. Dallas (TX), November 13–16, 2005.

32. Kadhiresan K, Carlson G. The role of implantable sensors for management of heart failure. Stud Health Technol Inform 2004;108:219–27.

33. Stevenson LW. Are hemodynamic goals viable in tailoring heart failure therapy? Hemodynamic goals are relevant. Controversies in cardiovascular medicine. Circulation 2006;113:1020–33.

34. Wadas TM. The implantable hemodynamic monitoring system. Crit Care Nurse 2005;25:14–26.

35. Magalski A, Adamson P, Gadler F, et al. Continuous ambulatory right heart pressure measurements with an implantable hemodynamic monitor: a multicenter 12-month follow-up study of patients with chronic heart failure. J Card Fail 2002;8:63–70.

36. Adamson PB, Conti JB, Smith AL, et al. Reducing events in patients with chronic heart failure (REDUCEhf) study design: continuous hemodynamic monitoring with an implantable defibrillator. Clin Cardiol 2007;30(11):567–75.

37. Ohlsson A, Kubo SH, Steinhaus D, et al. Continuous ambulatory monitoring of absolute right ventricular pressure and mixed venous oxygen saturation in patients with heart failure using an implantable hemodynamic monitor. Eur Heart J 2001;22:942–54.

38. Walton AS, Krum H. The HeartPOD implantable heart failure therapy system. Heart Lung Circ 2005; 14S:S31–3.

39. Tang WS. Collaboration among general cardiologists, heart failure specialists, and electrophysiologists: what are the barriers? Am J Cardiol 2007; 99(suppl):41G–4G.

40. AdvaMed. The Remote monitoring access act. Available at: http://www.advamed.org/MemberPortal/About/NewsRoom/NewsReleases/2006/09-13-2006_patientmonitoring.htm41. Accessed March 12, 2008.

Index

Note: Page numbers of article titles are in **boldface** type.

Heart Failure Clin 5 (2009) 279–282
doi:10.1016/S1551-7136(09)00009-9
1551-7136/09/$ – see front matter © 2009 Elsevier Inc. All rights reserved.

Moving?

Make sure your subscription moves with you!

To notify us of your new address, find your **Clinics Account Number** (located on your mailing label above your name), and contact customer service at:

E-mail: elspcs@elsevier.com

800-654-2452 (subscribers in the U.S. & Canada)
314-453-7041 (subscribers outside of the U.S. & Canada)

Fax number: 314-523-5170

Elsevier Periodicals Customer Service
11830 Westline Industrial Drive
St. Louis, MO 63146

*To ensure uninterrupted delivery of your subscription, please notify us at least 4 weeks in advance of move.

Printed and bound by CPI Group (UK) Ltd, Croydon, CR0 4YY

03/10/2024

01040355-0007